Introduction to Environmental Health

Daniel S. Blumenthal, M.D.

EDITOR

Springer Publishing Company
New York

Copyright © 1985 by Springer Publishing Company, Inc.

Springer Publishing Company, Inc.
536 Broadway
New York, New York 10012

85 86 87 88 89 / 10 9 8 7 6 5 4 3 2

Library of Congress Cataloging in Publication Data

Main entry under title:
Introduction to environmental health.
   Includes bibliographies and index.
   1. Environmental health.   I. Blumenthal, Daniel S. [DNLM: 1. Environmental Health.
WA 30 I613] RA565.I58   1985   616.9′8   84-23650
ISBN 0-8261-3900-0

Daniel S. Blumenthal, M.D., received his degree from the University of Chicago. He is professor and chairman in the Department of Community Medicine and Family Practice, Morehouse School of Medicine. He is a clinical assistant professor in the Departments of Community Health and Pediatrics at Emory University School of Medicine, Atlanta, Georgia.

Introduction to
Environmental Health

Contents

Preface

This book is designed primarily for students of medicine, nursing, and public health. It is intended to serve as a text for a general introductory course in environmental health and attempts to cover all major topic areas that are subsumed under the broad heading "environmental health." Its emphasis is on the impact of the environment on health, rather than ecological changes in the environment itself.

Environmental health is one of the oldest health-related disciplines, with roots in the study of sanitation and infectious disease epidemiology. Yet it is only in recent years that health professionals have gained an appreciation of the impact of the environment on a broad range of health problems. At the same time, the general public has become increasingly concerned with the effect on health of changes in the environment caused by humans. The popular press has helped to make places such as Love Canal, Three Mile Island, and Times Beach and the events associated with them a permanent part of the public consciousness.

Certainly, public concern with the effect of the environment on health has stimulated a great deal of research, and considerably more is known about environmental factors in disease etiology than was known only a few years ago. Still, there clearly are more questions than answers. If this book can motivate some readers to pursue answers to some of the questions and can stir others to pursue solutions to some of the known problems, it will have served its purpose well.

Thanks are due to Beverly Greene for editorial assistance and to Sheila Carson, Julia Blalock, and Pauletta Graves for secretarial assistance.

Contributors

Larry Auerbach received his M.B.A. from the University of Alabama and his J.D. from John Marshall Law School in Atlanta. He is a staff attorney with the Occupational Safety and Health Administration, Atlanta.

Herman T. Blumenthal received his M.D. and Ph.D. from Washington University, St. Louis, Missouri. He is an adjunct professor in the Department of Community Medicine, St. Louis University School of Medicine, and a research professor of gerontology, Washington University, St. Louis.

John Lewis Carden, Jr., received his Ph.D. in physical chemistry from Georgia Institute of Technology. He is an associate professor of health physics at Georgia Institute of Technology, Atlanta.

Keith M. Casto received his J.D. from Stetson University. He is a staff attorney with the Environmental Protection Agency, Atlanta.

D. Peter Drotman received his M.D. from the University of Southern California and his M.P.H. from UCLA. He is a medical epidemiologist with the Centers for Disease Control and is a clinical assistant professor in the Department of Community Health, Emory University School of Medicine, Atlanta.

Milford Greene received his Ph.D. from Wesleyan University in Middletown, Connecticut, and his M.P.H. from Harvard University. He is an associate professor of family and community medicine and Assistant Dean for Minority Affairs, Mercer University School of Medicine, Macon, Georgia.

Philip J. Landrigan received his M.D. from Harvard University and his M.Sc. from the London School of Tropical Medicine and Hygiene. He is Director of the Division of Surveillance, Hazard Evaluation, and Field Studies, National Institute of Occupational Safety and Health, Cincinnati, Ohio.

James M. Melius received his M.D. from the University of Illinois College of Medicine, Chicago, and his D.P.H. from the University of Illinois School of Public Health. He is Chief, Hazard Evaluation and Technical Assistance Branch, National Institute of Occupational Safety and Health, Cincinnati, Ohio.

Chapter 1

A Perspective on Environmental Health

Daniel S. Blumenthal

DEFINITION

What is "environmental health?" If one were to include in this term all factors in the human environment that affect health and every illness that has its etiology in the environment, then environmental health would encompass virtually all of health and medicine. Even genetic disease would be included, since many environmental factors may cause mutations and are thus responsible for some genetically transmitted conditions.

A more limited and more useful definition of environmental health as a discipline might be: the study of disease-causing agents that are introduced into the environment by humans, as well as the illnesses that are caused by these agents. This definition should not be interpreted strictly, for there are, to be sure, "natural" pollutants. Naturally occurring background radiation, for instance, may affect human health; toxins such as poisonous mushrooms may be found in nature and produce human disease; even pollens may constitute "natural air pollution" for hay-fever sufferers. Moreover, natural environmental factors such as climate and geography affect health status. But an approach that concentrates on environmental hazards of human origin is useful if for no other reason than that it encourages a focus on potentially remediable problems.

Environmental health as a discipline also implies a public health approach to disease and its agents rather than an approach at the level of the individual patient. This does not mean that the study of environmental health is unimportant to the clinician; on the contrary, it is essential that the health professional who cares for individuals be aware of environmental and other public health concerns and the impact that they may have on the patient. Unfortunately, it is common for clinicians to overlook the role of environmental and occupational exposures on the health of their patients, just as it is common for clinicians to overlook the public health importance of their own actions in, for instance, ordering radiologic studies.

The diagnosis and management of an illness in an individual is not generally considered part of the study of environmental health, however, even though the illness may have an environmental etiology. The focus of the discipline, is, rather, the study of pathogenic agents in the environment and their impact on populations and communities. Epidemiology thus becomes an important tool in this study.

Some areas of study are included in or excluded from the discipline of environmental health by convention. Thus, while foodstuffs are certainly part of the environment and are grown or prepared by humans, the study of nutrition is generally considered a separate discipline. Chemicals and other nonfood substances found in food are considered an environmental health concern, however, whether or not these substances are included intentionally as additives or are inadvertent contaminants.

Environmental factors of human origin that produce psychological stress have come to be recognized only recently as environmental health concerns; hence, intangibles such as noise and urban crowding—once considered to be within the domain of the social psychologist or the city planner—now also are scrutinized by the student of environmental health (Loring, 1974).

THE ROLE OF ENVIRONMENTAL HEALTH

If the 1960s were the decade of access to health care and the 1970s the decade of primary care, then it might be said that the 1980s are the decade of environmental health. The years 1960 through 1970 saw the growth of programs such as Medicare, Medicaid, and Neighborhood Health Centers, all of which were intended to provide most of the U.S. population with adequate access to health services. Between 1970 and 1980, public policy focused on encouraging the expansion of primary care services in order to promote the most appropriate health care for this now medically enfranchised population.

Most recently, however, we have begun to recognize that we are approaching the limits of the improvement in the health of the U.S. population that can be accomplished by individual health services. Indeed, each additional increment is achieved only at great cost: Expenditures on health care in this country are tripling every 10 years (Klarman, 1981), while health status is only inching upward.

At the same time, we have begun to recognize that many of the ills that continue to plague us have their roots in the environment. The only feasible approach to reducing morbidity from these problems is to attack their environmental roots. Cancer, for instance, is the second most frequent cause of death in the United States — and it has been estimated that 60 to 90 percent of cancers are environmentally caused (Hoover, 1979).

Whether or not one accepts estimates such as this, it is apparent that efforts at environmental improvement can have a positive effect in disease prevention. Other than immunization programs, there are few areas where there are similar opportunities for primary prevention.

CLASSES OF ENVIRONMENTAL HAZARDS

While there are hundreds of thousands of potential hazards in the environment, they can be lumped into fewer than a dozen classifications. A review of these will aid in bringing some organization to the study of environmental health.

1. *Infectious agents*. The control of epidemics of infectious disease is the traditional role of departments of public health. Such epidemics are often "environmental"; that is, they are the result of infectious agents introduced into the environment by humans through the water or food supplies. Mortality from infectious disease has been greatly reduced in this country in the last 50 years, and sanitation much improved, but food-borne and water-borne disease has by no means been eliminated. Over 10,000 cases of acute food-

borne disease (Centers for Disease Control [CDC], 1983) and up to 20,000 cases of acute water-borne disease (CDC, 1982) are reported annually in the United States, and the majority of cases remain unreported. Many fundamental sanitation problems remain: Unsafe water supplies and primitive means of sewage disposal are the rule in many rural communities, particularly in the Southeast.

2. *Irritants.* Sulfur dioxide (SO_2) and nitrogen dioxide (NO_2) are among the common respiratory irritants that pollute the air, particularly in urban areas. These substances can lead to rhinitis, pharyngitis, and bronchitis and can exacerbate preexisting respiratory disease. Other respiratory irritants are found in the occupational or domestic setting. Formaldehyde, for instance, is an irritant that is given off by urea formaldehyde foam insulation and has caused respiratory problems in residents of homes containing this type of insulation.

Skin irritants are largely an occupational problem; they are responsible for a variety of irritant rashes. Examples are chemical byproducts of certain manufacturing processes, such as sulfuric acid, and pesticides such as gamma benzene hexachloride.

3. *Respiratory fibrotic agents.* Dusts and fibers that are phagocytized and retained in the lung stimulate a fibrotic response and are responsible for a group of occupational pulmonary diseases known as pneumoconioses. These agents and the diseases they cause include coal dust (anthracosis, black lung); cotton dust (byssinosis, brown lung); cellulose (bagassosis, found in sugar cane workers); and asbestos (asbestosis). Metallic fumes, such as oxides of tin, iron, and beryllium, cause similar problems.

4. *Asphyxiants.* These are gases that prevent oxygen intake or prevent the utilization of oxygen by the body. The most notable example is carbon monoxide (CO), an air pollutant that is a component of automobile exhaust fumes. It also is found in some occupational settings and is emitted by faulty home heating units. Carbon monoxide combines with hemoglobin and blocks its ability to transport oxygen (Lisella, Johnson, & Holt, 1978).

5. *Allergens.* A variety of substances, including herbicides, insecticides, and some metals (particularly nickel), may trigger allergic responses in sensitized individuals. This is a particular problem in some occupational settings, where workers may develop allergies to substances with which they must work.

6. *Metabolic poisons.* Acute or chronic poisoning may result from many substances present in the environment. These include compounds that are manufactured as poisons, such as insecticides and herbicides; heavy metals such as lead, which is ubiquitous in the environment; and even substances such as fluoride that are beneficial in the proper dose but hazardous in overdose (CDC, 1980). Toxins may attack multiple sites or systems in the body or may be limited to a single site of action.

7. *Physical agents.* Trauma and accidents are the fourth most common cause of death in the United States and the leading cause among children and young adults (USDHHS, 1980). Accident control, therefore, is a very important environmental health concern. Perhaps the most important physical agent is the automobile; automobile accidents are the leading cause of accidental death. Homicide, occupational accidents, and accidents in the home are other leading problems.

Noise is another physical agent that deserves mention. In addition to its role as an agent of psychological stress, high noise levels can cause physical damage to hearing. This may be a particular problem in certain occupations (Gould & Sullivan, 1973).

8. *Psychological agents.* Stressful environmental conditions have become recognized contributors to both mental health problems and physical problems such as hypertension (Cassel, 1970). General environmental stresses such as urban noise and crowding have been mentioned already; perhaps of equal importance is occupational stress for executives; the assembly line worker who is under pressure to produce; and people in demanding, high-responsibility jobs such as air traffic controllers (Kasl, 1981).

9. *Mutagens.* Mutagenicity is the ability of an agent to alter genetic material. Mutagens include compounds such as vinyl chloride and dioxin, heavy metals such as cadmium, and ionizing radiation. The mutagenicity of an agent may be tested in the laboratory by cytogenetic studies on the white blood cells of exposed individuals, by examining cells of abortuses obtained from exposed women, by examining the cells of exposed animals, or by introducing the agent into bacterial test systems (de Serres, 1979).

In humans and other higher-order animals, mutations (alterations of single genes) are rarely identified as stemming from an environmental exposure. The result of exposure to a mutagen is more likely to be a birth defect or a cancer. Hence, mutagenicity is generally a laboratory determination; mutagenic agents generally manifest themselves as carcinogens or teratogens.

   10. *Teratogens.* As just noted, some agents, such as radiation, dioxin, and cadmium, may cause birth defects by altering genetic material. Others — such as the notorious drug thalidomide — may cause abnormalities of organogenesis.

   11. *Carcinogens.* The extent of the hazard to human health caused by chemical carcinogens in the environment is presently the subject of considerable debate. In fact, the problem may be suffering from overexposure in the popular media: When it begins to seem that "everything causes cancer," people become apathetic. Actually, no more than about 10 percent of the 10,000 or so chemicals in the environment are carcinogenic. Some — such as cigarette smoke, asbestos, and vinyl chloride — are well known. Others are obscure. Interestingly, the first known chemical carcinogen — soot — was identified as long ago as 1775, by Sir Percival Pott, as the cause of scrotal cancer in chimney sweeps (Pott, 1775).

HOST–AGENT INTERACTIONS

   Many substances have multiple potential effects on the human body, as shown in Table 1-1. The manifestation in an individual of exposure to an environmental hazard is determined by the interactions of agent, host, and environmental factors. *Agent* factors include the inherent properties of the agent as well as its dose. *Host* factors include the portal of entry of the agent (oral, skin, respiratory) as well as the host's individual susceptibility to the agent. This susceptibility is determined by immune status, nutritional status, heredity, and a host of unknown or little-understood factors. *Environmental* factors — other than the presence of the agent itself — may include the concurrent presence of other hazardous agents or factors affecting the host's resistance.

   Of particular interest is the fate of environmental chemicals after they enter the body. Four possibilities deserve special mention:

   1. *Metabolism.* Many toxic substances are detoxified in the body by a variety of enzymatic processes, most of which take place

Table 1-1 Known and Suspected Effects of Some Environmental Hazards

	Irritant	Pulmonary Fibrotic Agent	Metabolic Poison	Mutagen	Teratogen	Carcinogen
Fibers						
Asbestos		X				X
Cotton Dust		X				
Organic Chemicals						
Gamma-Benzene Hexachloride (insecticide)	X		X			
2,4,5-T (herbicide)	X		X	X	X	
Vinyl Chloride Monomer			X			X
Heavy Metals						
Cadmium			X			X
Lead			X			
Radiation	X	X	X	X	X	X

in the liver. The ability of the body to perform these transformations makes a number of potentially dangerous chemicals useful as drugs. Obviously, liver disease, enzyme deficiencies, or other conditions that reduce the body's ability to carry out these metabolic processes increase the individual's susceptibility to the toxic effects of these chemicals.

On the other hand, some apparently harmless substances are metabolized to become toxic agents. In fact, the majority of chemical carcinogens are actually procarcinogens that acquire the ability to cause cancer only after enzymatic transformation to a related compound (Farber, 1981). In some cases, more than one step is required. For example, nitrites (found in cured meats) and amines (found in many foods and chemicals) may combine in the gastrointestinal tract to form nitrosamines, which are considered carcinogenic. Actually, nitrosamines are procarcinogens that are converted, by enzymatic oxidation, to carcinogenic alkylating moieties.

2. *Excretion.* Most chemicals that are introduced into the body are excreted subsequently, sometimes in unchanged form, but more often as a metabolized byproduct. Most excretion is accomplished by the kidneys. Some substances may be excreted through the lungs (carbon tetrachloride), gastrointestinal tract (heavy metals), or even sweat, saliva, or milk (Lippman & Schlesinger, 1979). Obviously, disease affecting the kidneys or other excretory organs will diminish the body's ability to rid itself of hazardous chemicals.

3. *Storage.* Some substances are neither metabolized nor excreted by the body but are, at least in part, retained in their original state. They may be mobilized later as a result of known or unknown factors, thus presenting the body with a sudden large load of the substance. Lead, which is stored in bone, is an example. Children who have consumed small amounts of lead in the form of chips of lead-based paint over a considerable period of time may suddenly become acutely toxic. This occurs most often in the summer; it is thought that sunlight may play a role in mobilizing the lead stores (Chisolm & Kaplan, 1968).

Other examples which are causing current concern are chemicals which are stored in fat, such as polychlorinated biphenyls (PCBs) (Wickizer, Brilliant, Copeland, & Tilden, 1981) and DDT (Woodard, Ferguson, & Wilson, 1976). In the lactating mother, stored fat is mobilized and the chemicals may be released in the milk and transmitted to the nursing infant.

4. *Synergism and promotion.* As a result of mechanisms that are poorly understood, the whole risk of cancer in some cases may be greater than the sum of its parts. That is, an individual exposed to two carcinogens simultaneously may be at greater risk of cancer than would be calculated from the two agents' combined individual probabilities of causing cancer (synergism). Alternatively, a relatively weak carcinogen may become a relatively strong one in the presence of a noncarcinogen (promotion) (Farber, 1981).

A well-known example of synergism is the combined effect of asbestos exposure and cigarette smoking. In the study by Hammond, Selikoff, and Seidman (1979), nonsmoking asbestos workers were about five times as likely to die from lung cancer as persons in a nonsmoking, non-asbestos-worker control group (Table 1–2). Smokers who were not exposed to asbestos were 10 times as likely to die of lung cancer as the control group. If the risk of cancer from cigarette smoke were added to the risk from asbestos, an asbestos worker who smoked would have 15 times the risk of death from lung cancer, compared to a person exposed to neither carcinogen. In reality, asbestos workers who smoked were found to have over 53 times the lung cancer risk of the controls (i.e., a relative risk of 53). Thus, asbestos and cigarette smoke (or some component of it) are synergistic: The cancer risk from exposure to the two agents

Table 1–2   Lung Cancer Death Rates and Mortality Ratios in Smoking and Nonsmoking Asbestos Workers and Controls

Group	Death Rate[a]	Mortality Ratio[b]
Control (nonsmokers)	11.3	1.00
Asbestos Workers (nonsmokers)	58.4	5.17
Control (smokers)	122.6	10.85
Asbestos Workers (smokers)	601.6	53.24

[a]Rates per 100,000 person-years standardized for age on the distribution of the person-years of all the asbestos workers.

[b] $\dfrac{\text{Death Rate}}{\text{Death Rate for Control (nonsmokers)}} = \text{Mortality Ratio}$

Source: Data from E. C. Hammond, I. J. Selikoff, and H. Seidman. Asbestos Exposure, Cigarette Smoking, and Death Rates. *Annals of the New York Academy of Sciences*, 1979, *330*, 473–490.

together is greater than the combined risks of the individual agents.

(Viewed another way, either the smoking or nonsmoking asbestos worker has 5 times the lung cancer risk of his counterpart [smoking or nonsmoking] who does not work with asbestos. The study should not be interpreted to mean that working with asbestos is safe if the worker does not smoke.)

Agents of the second mechanism, promotion, generally have been identified in animal studies. Certain components of croton oil (phorbol esters), for instance, have been found to be potent promoters of mouse skin tumors after exposure to dimethylbenzanthracene or other carcinogens (Hecker, 1978).

Considerations of synergism and promotion are likely to assume greater importance as we learn more about carcinogens in the environment and their relationship to human cancers. Substances that presently are thought to be of little importance because their carcinogenicity is weak in animal studies may take on greater significance if we learn that they act synergistically with other environmental compounds or if their cancer-causing potential is enhanced by environmental promoters.

ENTRY OF POLLUTANTS INTO THE ENVIRONMENT

Public concern with the effects of hazardous agents in the environment has led to continual reexamination of the mechanisms by which these agents enter the environment and the measures that can be taken to limit their entry. The specific measures to be taken obviously are dependent on the mode of entry of the agent into the environment. Often, however, the problem boils down to one of setting standards. The agencies responsible for limiting environmental hazards (Environmental Protection Agency, Occupational Safety and Health Administration, local health departments, etc.) must take into consideration known information about the toxicity of the agent in question, available or potentially available technology for limiting its entry into the environment, the societal importance of the industry or process of which it is a byproduct, the cost of limiting its entry, and a variety of political factors. The standards that result are often a compromise and sometimes may appear irrational when considered only from the perspective of health. For instance, permissible exposure levels to cotton dust for workers in different sectors of the cotton industry range from 200 μg/m^3 of air to 750 μg/m^3, even though it is likely that workers in all sectors of the industry have the same average susceptibility to byssinosis.

There are four basic ways in which hazardous substances may enter the environment and be transmitted to humans:

1. *Direct exposure to the source.* This mechanism is of great importance in occupational settings, where the population exposed is relatively small but exposure levels may be high.

Persons also are exposed directly when hazards are introduced intentionally into the environment as consumer products — usually before their hazardous nature is known. Examples include lead in paint, Tris flame retardant in children's sleepwear (later found to be carcinogenic), and DDT.

Direct exposure also may be considered the means by which individuals are exposed to agents of physical trauma. Again, the population exposed to a particular source is small, but the "exposure level" may be high.

2. *Direct discharge into air or water.* Until relatively recent years, industrial waste products generally were discharged directly into the environment through smokestacks or into a convenient river or stream. Similarly, untreated sewage was discharged into rivers by municipalities, and automobile exhausts were uncontrolled. The diluting effect of the air or water was thought to render the hazardous discharges safe.

The environmental hazards posed by these practices are more greatly appreciated now, of course, and the discharges are relatively easy to detect at their source. The controversy — as described previously — relates to the standards that must be set for regulating the treatment of the discharges before their release and for acceptable concentrations of hazardous substances in the environment.

3. *Inadequate landfills.* A landfill is a site for the disposal of waste (either "hazardous" — chemical or nuclear — or "sanitary") on land. Landfills are engineered to prevent the escape of pollutants into the environment. Containing the waste successfully may pose a difficult challenge, particularly if the substances in question are stable chemicals that may persist unchanged indefinitely or nuclear wastes with half lives of hundreds or thousands of years. In the event that a landfill (or similar disposal site) is inadequate, pollutants may enter the human environment by runoff and leaching or through the food chain.

      a. *Runoff*. Rain may carry hazardous substances away from the landfill site to surface water (rivers and lakes) that is used for human consumption; thus, the relationship of landfills to bodies of surface water is an important consideration.

      b. *Leaching*. Rainwater percolating through the landfill may carry hazardous substances downward to enter an aquifer (a body of ground water). At a site somewhat remote from the landfill, the aquifer may be tapped via a well for drinking purposes. Hence, considerations in locating landfills include the relationship of the proposed site to aquifers that are or might be used by humans, and the permeability of the soil separating the landfill from the ground water beneath.

      c. *Travel through the food chain*. Pollutants in the environment may not be consumed directly by humans as they would had they entered the drinking water supply through runoff or leaching. Instead, the hazardous substances may be incorporated into plants, which are eaten by small animals, which are eaten by larger animals, which are, in turn, eaten by humans. Thus, polychlorinated biphenyls that have run off into bodies of fresh water eventually find their way into fish that serve as human food.

    4. *Dumping*. Recent environmental history is replete with "horror stories" of large quantities of toxic chemicals that have been dumped, willy-nilly, into the environment. These include the "Valley of the Drums" in Kentucky, in which 17,000 chemical-filled drums were littered about a seven-acre site 25 miles south of Louisville; the Byron, Illinois, incident in which 1,500 drums filled with chemical waste were buried for an unknown number of years, leaking cyanide, heavy metals, and other toxins into both surface and ground water; the notorious "Love Canal" episode; and many others (US Environmental Protection Agency, 1980). Unfortunately, these incidents are not merely historical footnotes. Illegal dumping of haz-

ardous wastes continues, since it is cheaper and easier than conform- *RCRA 1976*
ing to the requirements of the Resource Conservation and Recovery
Act (RCRA) of 1976, which regulates disposal of chemical wastes
(Kovacs & Klucsik, 1977). Under cover of night, tank trucks may
discharge their contents through manholes into urban sewer systems
or into ravines in rural areas. Such "horror stories" will continue
to find their way into the daily papers.

ENVIRONMENTAL EPIDEMIOLOGY

As indicated at the outset of this chapter, environmental health
implies a public health approach almost by definition. Environmental hazards are dispersed throughout populations or communities
and must be studied in their relationship to these groups. The methods that must be used are those of epidemiology, which is defined
as "the study of the distribution and determinants of diseases and
injuries in human populations" (Mausner & Bahn, 1974).

It has been said that epidemiology is not a science in itself, but
rather a set of tools that can be applied to a variety of disciplines.
These tools have been used extensively in the field of environmental health; in fact, it is probable that most known environmental
toxins and the extent of the damage that they cause have been identified by the epidemiological process.

The purpose of epidemiology is to discover the cause of disease
so that it can be prevented. Having said this, one also must acknowl-
edge that causality can never be proven by epidemiological methods. *supposed*
Epidemiology can establish an *association* between a putative cause
and a disease, but association does not prove causality. For instance,
it can be shown (as described earlier in this chapter) that asbestos
workers are five times more likely than non-asbestos workers to contract lung cancer. This association does not prove scientifically that
asbestos causes lung cancer, however. First, there is a small but cal-
culable probability that the association is due merely to chance variation in the distribution of lung cancer victims in the population.
Second, it is at least theoretically possible that some substance in
asbestos mills other than the asbestos itself — or some other factor
common to asbestos workers — is actually the cause of lung cancer.

Despite these caveats regarding "proof," a strong, consistent, and specific association between an agent and a disease that occurs following exposure to that agent is generally accepted as sufficient grounds to act as if there were a cause-and-effect relationship (on the other hand, a weak relationship may be seen merely as grounds for "exercising caution" or calling for further studies).

The remainder of this chapter will be devoted to a brief, superficial overview of some of the basic concepts and methods of epidemiology. For a more thorough discussion, the reader is referred to any of the several excellent epidemiology textbooks available.

Rates

In epidemiology, data most often are expressed as rates, particularly when comparisons are to be made between two different populations. A rate is a ratio between two numbers in which the denominator represents a population at risk and the numerator represents some part of that population. Frequently, a rate is expressed with a standardized denominator, that is, the number of cases of a condition per (for instance) 1000 people.

An *incidence rate* refers to the rate of occurrence of *new* cases during a defined period of time, while a *prevalence rate* refers to all *current* cases — both old and new — at a point in time (*point prevalence*) or over a period of time (*period prevalence*). These two kinds of rates should not be confused.

Rates may need to be adjusted to compensate for age differences (or, occasionally, other differences) between two populations. If, for instance, the mortality rate in a retirement community were compared with that of a typical suburb, the rate probably would be higher in the former. It would be erroneous to attribute the difference to some environmental cause, however. Since the population of the retirement community would be older than that of the suburb, it would be expected to have a higher mortality rate. To identify a true difference between the two communities, the rates should be age adjusted; that is, the age distribution of the two populations should be converted to that of some standard population and the mortality rates recalculated accordingly. (Without adjustment, the rates are called crude mortality rates).

Sources of Morbidity and Mortality Data

The concept of surveillance is an important one in epidemiology. Surveillance is "the continuing scrutiny of all aspects of occurrence and spread of disease that are pertinent to effective control" (Benenson, 1980). Certain infectious diseases (e.g., salmonellosis, shigellosis, trichinosis) as well as a few noninfectious diseases (e.g., lead poisoning) must be reported, by law, to state health departments. State data then are forwarded to the federal Centers for Disease Control, which publish it weekly.

Information on all births, deaths, and fetal deaths — in the form of birth and death certificates — also is collected at the state level. Although this is not usually termed surveillance, it fits the definition, and death certificates are the source of a great deal of data used in epidemiological studies. Caution must be used in interpreting death-certificate data, however, for the kind of diagnostic information recorded on a death certificate may vary considerably according to the jurisdiction collecting the certificate or the doctor filling it out.

The collection of data on other conditions differs from state to state. Some states maintain cancer registries; others conduct surveillance over such conditions as inborn errors of metabolism and childhood anemia. Agencies other than the health department keep records on health-related events such as automobile fatalities and homicides.

Surveillance programs, which collect data on new events, permit the calculation of incidence (rather than prevalence) rates. The denominators for these rates are usually census data. A national census is taken every 10 years, and significant population shifts may take place during the intervening decade. Thus, these figures, like those derived from death certificates, must be used cautiously.

Often an investigator wishes to obtain information concerning a condition on which surveillance data are not maintained or may be inadequate. In this case, a survey is done. Usually, a survey will involve less than the entire population at risk (unless this population is relatively small), so a representative sample must be chosen. Statistical methods are available for determining the size of the sample that should be chosen at random; that is, every member of the population at risk should have an equal probability of being selected. Bias is likely to result if subjects are self-selected (that is, if they volunteer to participate or are chosen from, say, among hospital or clinic patients).

Since a survey generally will detect all persons with the condition under study at a point in time, this method usually provides point prevalence data. A survey could provide incidence data, however, if subjects were asked about the onset of disease during the past month or year.

Types of Epidemiology

Epidemiologic methods may be grouped under one of three headings: descriptive, analytic, or experimental.

Descriptive Epidemiology. Descriptive epidemiology is the study of the amount and distribution of a disease within a population by time, place, and personal characteristics (Mausner & Bahn, 1974). The personal characteristics studied in describing disease patterns usually include the age, race, and sex of the subjects and may include other factors such as occupation, socioeconomic status, type of housing occupied, and even religion. The fact that several victims of a rare cancer, angiosarcoma of the liver, shared a common occupational exposure led to the general recognition of vinyl chloride as a carcinogen (Block, 1974).

The time distribution of an illness may provide significant clues to its etiology. The temporal relationship of air pollution episodes to outbreaks of acute respiratory disease, for instance, has helped identify some of the health problems associated with air pollution (Whittemore & Korn, 1980).

The geographic distribution of a disease also may provide valuable information. Analysis of cancer mortality rates, for instance, shows that the highest U.S. rates occur around major urban industrial centers, particularly in the northeast, and in the lower Mississippi River Valley — places where people may be exposed to relatively high concentrations of pollutants (Hoover, 1979).

Analytic Epidemiology. Descriptive epidemiology often leads to a hypothesis regarding the cause of the disease under study. Analytic epidemiology is the process by which this hypothesis is tested and implies a search for association between disease occurrence and possible causative influence (Fox, Hall, & Elveback, 1970). There are three basic types of analytic studies: retrospective, prospective, and historical prospective.

1. *Retrospective (Case Control) Study.* In this type of study, persons with an illness (cases) are identified and compared with a control group of persons who share as many personal characteristics as possible with the cases, but who do not have the disease. The two groups then are compared for the presence or absence of suspected causes of the disease ("risk factors"). A retrospective study starts with the effect (disease) and attempts to discover a cause. For instance, a group of lung cancer patients might be compared with a group of healthy controls (matched for age, race, and sex) for a history of cigarette smoking.

Retrospective studies have several advantages. As compared with prospective studies (described later), they are quicker, easier, and less expensive to perform. Smaller numbers of subjects are required for retrospective studies, and they are more suitable for studying rare diseases. On the other hand, they may be biased (inaccurate) because they depend on memory or after-the-fact data: Subjects may be asked to recall risk factors to which they were exposed many years ago. For this reason, prospective studies, while more difficult to perform, generally are considered more valid.

2. *Prospective (Cohort) Study.* In this type of study, a group (cohort) of persons that is exposed to a suspected cause of disease is matched with a group that is not so exposed. Both groups are followed over time and observed for the occurrence of the disease under study. This type of study, then, starts with the cause (or suspected cause) and works toward the effect. For instance, a group of smokers and a group of nonsmokers, matched for age, race, and sex, might be followed and observed for the occurrence of lung cancer.

This type of study is superior to a retrospective study in that actual exposure to the risk factor can be documented carefully. Moreover, the study results will provide information on the incidence of the disease in question in exposed and nonexposed individuals. However, it may be much more expensive and time consuming than a retrospective study; in the smoking-and-cancer study suggested, the cohorts might have to be followed for 20 to 40 years.

3. *Historical Prospective (Retrospective Cohort or Nonconcurrent Cohort) Study.* This type of study might be considered a cross between a prospective and a retrospective study; it combines some of the advantages and some of the disadvantages of each. A cohort of individuals whose exposure to a risk factor was established at some time in the past is compared with another cohort, which has not been so exposed, for the occurrence of disease. For instance, a group of smokers over 45 years old might be compared with a group of nonsmokers of the same age for the occurrence of lung cancer. Similarly, the cancer incidence in asbestos workers and non-asbestos workers might be compared, or the incidence of cancer or some other disease examined in residents of two different counties where environmental exposures are different. As in the other types of studies, both groups of individuals should be matched as closely as possible for age, race, sex, and other personal characteristics.

Since this is a type of cohort study, it starts with the suspected cause and works toward the effect. It is relatively quick and inexpensive, like a retrospective study, and provides incidence data, like a prospective study. On the other hand, it shares with the retrospective study the disadvantage of depending on memory or data collected for some other purpose to determine risk-factor exposure levels.

Experimental Epidemiology.   Descriptive and analytic epidemiologic studies use information that is generated naturally and merely collected and analyzed by the epidemiologist. In experimental epidemiology, however, the environment of the subject is manipulated by the experimenter and the results of these manipulations studied.

Therapeutic trials, in which an experimental drug is administered to one group of individuals suffering from a disease while a placebo is given to another, is a type of experimental epidemiology (note that these are prospective studies). Experiments have been done in which suspected infectious or allergenic agents have been administered to volunteers to test for disease causation. Obviously, though, ethical considerations prevent human-subject testing of suspected carcinogens or teratogens in this manner.

Typically, suspected chemical carcinogens are tested in rats, mice, and sometimes hamsters of both sexes. Once the maximally tolerated dose (MTD) of the chemical is determined, groups of 50 male and 50 female rodents are given the MTD and half the MTD in a two-year test, or sometimes a lifetime test. Postmortem studies of the animals then are conducted and the incidence of tumors in the experimental animals compared with that of a control group. Such tests, as presently conducted, may cost $300,000 to $500,000 (Weisburger & Williams, 1981).

These experiments have led to some of the most controversial findings in the field of environmental health, and many of these controversies have been debated in the halls of Congress and in the lay press. These debates stem from the fact that the MTDs are far larger, on a per-weight basis, than the dose to which humans are likely to be exposed. For instance, the popular sugar substitute, saccharin, has been found to be carcinogenic in animals; but, in order to consume a dose of saccharin equivalent to that administered to the experimental animals, a human would have to drink over a case of diet soda daily.

There are two reasons for using very large doses of suspected carcinogens in animal experiments. First, the latent period (the time from first exposure to a carcinogen, to the development of a cancer) for most cancers in humans is on the order of 20 to 40 years. Most experimental animals, however, have life expectancies of only a few years; therefore, large doses of suspected carcinogens are administered to the animals in the hope of shortening the latent period.

Second, a weak carcinogen administered in a relatively small dose to the 200 or so rodents that are used in a standard test might not cause any of the animals to develop cancer. In order to produce a statistically valid demonstration of the carcinogenicity of an agent that causes one cancer in every 10,000 exposed individuals (people or rats), for instance, it would be necessary to test the agent in 30,000 rats (USDHEW, 1977). Such a test would be prohibitively expensive, particularly considering the thousands of chemicals that must be tested. It is obviously important to define the cancer-causing potential of even weak carcinogens, however, if they are widespread in the environment. An agent such as that suggested, which causes a cancer incidence of 1/10,000 exposed persons, if present in the environment of (or consumed by) 10 million people, would cause 1000 cases of cancer.

Newer strategies in testing for carcinogenesis may permit the use of relatively rapid, relatively inexpensive tests — such as *in vitro* tests for mutagenicity — as preliminary assays. The more time consuming and expensive *in vivo* studies then may be reserved for the more highly suspect chemicals.

Political and Social Considerations

The trade-offs involved in attempting to limit health hazards in the environment are many and complex. Some of these are scientific. Tetraethyl lead now is being phased out as a component of gasoline because of the dangers of polluting the atmosphere with lead from automobile exhaust fumes. One of the replacements for organic lead in gasoline is organic manganese; however, the health effects of organic manganese are not well understood (Joselow, Tobias, Koehler, et al., 1978). It is possible that in attempting a solution to one problem, we have created another. This, of course, is not a unique example; the pesticide literature is replete with others.

Some trade-offs are political. The laws and regulations that are intended to limit environmental and occupational health hazards are compromises that are formulated only after long and intense debate and lobbying. Repeatedly, the extent of the danger posed by a putative health hazard is weighed against the technological and economic consequences of regulating it.

What is to be the role of the scientist in these debates? Some observers perhaps would suggest that the scientist should only provide the data upon which political compromises can be forged. An alternative approach, however, might be to treat the community as a patient. Just as the physician urges a patient to eliminate personal health hazards such as tobacco or alcohol abuse, so might the physician or basic scientist advocate in the community or at the legislative level for elimination of environmental health hazards.

REFERENCES

Benenson, A (ed) (1980): *Control of Communicable Disease In Man, 13th ed.* Washington, DC: American Public Health Association.

Block, JB (1974): Angiosarcoma of the Liver Following Vinyl Chloride Exposure. *JAMA* 229:53–54.

Cassel, J (1970): Physical Illness in Response to Stress. In Levine, S, and Scotch, NA (eds): *Social Stress.* Chicago: Aldine.

Centers for Disease Control (1982): *Water-related Disease Outbreaks Surveillance. Annual Summary 1981.* DHHS Publication No. (CDC) 82-8385.

Centers for Disease Control (1983): *Foodborne Disease Surveillance. Annual Summary 1979.* DHHS Publication No. (CDC) 83-8185.

Chisolm, JJ, and Kaplan, E (1968): Lead Poisoning in Childhood—Comprehensive Management and Prevention. *J Peds* 73:942-950.

deSerres, FJ (1979): Evaluation of Tests for Mutagenicity as Indicators of Environmental Mutagens and Carcinogens. *Ann NY Acad Sci* 329:75-84.

Farber, E (1981): Chemical Carcinogenesis. *New Eng J Med* 23:1379-1389.

Fox, JP, Hall, CE, and Elveback, LR (1970): *Epidemiology: Man and Disease.* New York: Macmillan.

Gould, WJ, and Sullivan, RF (1973): Noise. *Ann NY Acad Sci* 216:17-30.

Hammond, EC, Selikoff, IJ, and Seidman, H (1979): Asbestos Exposure, Cigarette Smoking, and Death Rates. *Ann NY Acad Sci* 33:473-492.

Hecker, E (1978): Biochemical Mechanism of Tumor Promotion. In Slaga, TJ, Sivak, A, and Boutwell, RK (eds): *Mechanisms of Tumor Promotion and Co-carcinogenesis.* Vol 2. New York: Raven Press.

Hoover, R (1979): Environmental Cancer. *Ann NY Acad Sci* 329:50-60.

Joselow, M, Tobias, E, Koehler, R, et al. (1978): Manganese Pollution in the City Environment and its Relationship to Traffic Density. *Am J Pub Health* 68:557-560.

Kasl, SV (1981): The Challenge of Studying the Disease Effects of Stressful Work Conditions. *Am J Pub Health* 71:682-684.

Klarman, NE (1981): Health Care Financing. In Clark, DW, and MacMahon, B. *Preventive and Community Medicine.* Boston: Little, Brown.

Kovacs, WL, and Klucsik (1977): The New Federal Role in Solid Waste Management: The Resource Conservation and Recovery Act of 1976. *Columbia J Env Law* 3:205-261.

Lippman, M, and Schlesinger, RB (1979): Chemical Contamination in the Human Environment. New York: Oxford University Press.

Lisella, FS, Johnson, W, and Holt, K (1978): Mortality from Carbon Monoxide in Georgia, 1961-1973. *J Med Assoc Ga* (Feb):98-100.

Loring, WC (1974): Social Psychological Indicators for Planning Man's Environment. Proceedings of the Environmental Planning Seminar, Drexel University, Philadelphia.

Mausner, J, and Bahn, A (1974): *Epidemiology: An Introductory Text.* Philadelphia: WB Saunders.

Pott, P (1775): Chirurgical Observations Relative to the Cancer of the Scrotum. Reprinted in *Nat Cancer Inst Monogr* (1963) 10:7-13.

U.S. Department of Health, Education and Welfare (1977): *Basic Concepts of Environmental Health.* Public Health Service, NIH, National Institute of Environment Health Science. DHEW Publication No. (NIH) 77-1254.

U.S. Department of Health and Human Services (1980): *Health United States 1980.* Hyattsville, Md.: USDHHS Publication No. (PHS) 81-1232.

U.S. Environmental Protection Agency (1980): Everybody's Problem: Hazardous Waste. Washington, DC.: Office of Water and Waste Management, Publication No. SW-826.

Weisburger, JH, and Williams GM (1981): Carcinogen Testing: Current Problems and New Approaches. *Science* 214:401–407.

Whittemore, AS, and Korn, EL (1980): Asthma and Air Pollution in the Los Angeles Area. *Am J Pub Health* 70:687–697.

Wickizer, TM, Brilliant, LB, Copeland, R, and Tilden, R (1981): Polychlorinated Biphenyl Contamination of Nursing Mothers' Milk in Michigan. *Am J Pub Health* 71:132–138.

Woodard, BT, Ferguson, BB, and Wilson, DJ (1976): DDT Levels in Milk of Rural Indigent Blacks. *Am J Dis Child* 130:400–403.

Chapter 2

Infectious Agents in the Environment

Daniel S. Blumenthal

Environmentally transmitted infectious disease constitutes the oldest environmental health problem of humanity. In the United States in recent years, manufactured toxins and carcinogens have generated widespread concern; however, in the nonindustrialized parts of the world, infectious disease, much of it environmentally transmitted, remains by far the greatest cause of morbidity and mortality, as it has since ancient times. Moreover, in this country, environmental spread of infectious disease has by no means been eliminated. Thousands of cases of food- and water-borne illness — and even soil-borne parasitic infections — still occur each year.

Infectious disease is considered to be environmentally transmitted when it is spread from a common source (usually food, water, or soil); or by a vector; or occasionally by fomites. Strictly speaking, infections transmitted from person to person by droplet or aerosol might be considered to be spread through the environment. However, such illnesses usually cannot be controlled by environmental manipulations and are thus not generally classified as environmental health concerns.

Infectious disease spread through the environment has been described in some of humanity's earliest writings. Schistosomiasis, a water-borne illness, was known in ancient Egypt. Plague, spread by vector, appears in the writings of Dionysius in the third century;

the first pandemic of this disease was documented in the sixth century.

The mode of transmission of these illnesses, of course, was not known until relatively recent times. John Snow, the English physician, is credited with first documenting environmental spread of a disease when he demonstrated in the early 1850s that cholera in London was transmitted through drinking water. Snow, however, knew nothing of the microbial nature of infectious disease; he attributed cholera to the consumption of "water containing the sewage of London, and, amongst it, whatever might have come from the cholera patients . . ." (Snow, 1855). Pasteur and Koch later demonstrated the role of microbes in the etiology of infectious disease.

Communicable disease control was the original mission of state and local health departments in the United States, and infectious disease is today the only environmental health hazard whose control is vested primarily with state and local officials. Laws and regulations concerning environmental toxins and carcinogens and occupational health hazards are primarily a function of the federal government; but the power to create and enforce sanitary codes remains in the hands of state and local officials.

WATER-BORNE INFECTIOUS DISEASE

The provision of sanitary water supplies to the bulk of the world's population remains one of the great public health challenges. The annual death and disability of hundreds of thousands of people in the developing countries from water-borne infections such as schistosomiasis, dracunculiasis, and the diarrheal diseases has led the World Health Organization to declare the 1980s the International Clean Water Decade. This declaration includes the difficult goal of attaining safe water sources for all by 1990.

In the United States, sanitary drinking water supplies often are taken for granted, yet over 30,000 rural communities in this country (not including isolated single residences) do not have safe central water systems. In 1981, 32 outbreaks of water-borne disease, affecting 4430 persons, were reported to the federal Centers for Disease Control; in 1980, there were 50 outbreaks affecting 20,008 people (CDC, 1982). These numbers represent only the proverbial tip of the iceberg, for the great majority of outbreaks remain unreported. An outbreak of water-borne illness may or may not come to the attention of state or local health officials, depending on the size of the outbreak, the interest of local physicians, and the investigative resources of the health department.

Water Supplies

Drinking water may be obtained from either surface sources (lakes and streams) or underground sources; the former are more likely to be contaminated with infectious organisms.

Water Purification.   A variety of processes is used to treat municipal water supplies. Sand filtration and chlorination virtually eliminate bacteria from the water. Other processes, such as chemical coagulation, sedimentation, aeration, and ion exchange, are used to remove particulate matter, minerals, and gases (McGauhey, 1968). Water supplies serving smaller groups of people or individual residences may be simply chlorinated or even untreated.

The cleanliness of water is ascertained by performing coliform counts, a procedure in which the water is cultured and the number of fecal coliform bacteria present — mainly *Escherichia coli* — is determined. Although the fecal coliforms so measured may not be pathogenic, they often are associated with pathogens and thus are used as indicators of probable water safety. Coliform counts commonly are expressed as Most Probable Number of bacteria per 100 ml (MPN/100 ml) of water. Federal regulations state that raw water to be purified for municipal use should contain no more than 20 MPN/100 ml; the coliform count of treated water should be zero (U.S. Environmental Protection Agency, 1976). Some agents of disease, such as chemicals and *Giardia* cysts, may be present in treated water even in the absence of fecal coliforms.

An additional test sometimes applied to drinking water is the free chlorine residual determination, which measures the adequacy of chlorination.

Drinking water may be contaminated with infectious organisms because (1) the water is untreated; (2) deficiencies are present in the treatment system; (3) deficiencies exist in the distribution system, such as a cross-connection between sewage and water lines; or (4) a properly functioning treatment system is unable to remove contaminating agents such as *Giardia* cysts or chemicals.

Types of Water Systems and Outbreaks.   The Safe Drinking Water Act of 1974 (PL93-523) defines three types of water systems. *Municipal systems* serve large or small communities, subdivisions, or trailer parks of at least 15 service connections or 25 year-round residents. *Semipublic systems* are those in institutions, industries, camps, parks, or service stations that may be used by the general public. *Individual systems* (generally wells and springs) are those used by single or several residences or by persons traveling outside populated areas, such as backpackers.

Most outbreaks of water-borne disease in this country involve semipublic water systems (see Table 2-1), and most of these occur during the summer (see Figure 2-1). Treatment deficiencies and the use of untreated ground water account for the great majority of these episodes. These epidemiologic data point up the fact that water systems serving campgrounds and parks are the greatest cause of reported water-borne disease outbreaks in the United States. The influx of visitors to these areas during the summer places considerable stress on small treatment units and exposes large numbers of people to untreated or inadequately treated water.

Outbreaks involving municipal water systems, while reported less often than those related to semipublic systems, account for a greater number of cases because of the large number of people af-

Table 2-1   Water-borne Disease Outbreaks, by Type of System and System Deficiency, 1971–1978

Cause	Number of Outbreaks				
	Municipal	Semipublic	Individual	Total	(%)
Untreated surface water	8	8	10	26	(12)
Untreated ground water	7	54	11	72	(32)
Treatment deficiency	22	51	0	73	(33)
Deficiency in distribution system	26	7	1	34	(15)
Miscellaneous	5	10	4	19	(8)
TOTAL	68 (30%)	130 (58%)	26 (12%)	224	(100)

Figure 2-1   Outbreaks of Waterborne Diseases, by Month, United States, 1971–1978

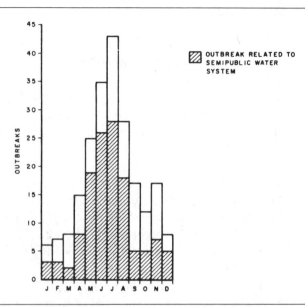

Source: Centers for Disease Control. *Water-related Disease Surveillance, Annual Summary, 1978.* Atlanta: CDC, 1980, USDHHS pub. no. (CDC) 80-8385.
Unshaded areas represent outbreaks related to municipal or individual water systems.

fected in some urban outbreaks. Defects in treatment units and distribution systems are responsible for most of these episodes (see Table 2–1).

Disease Related to Recreational Water Use

Illness caused by swimming or bathing in contaminated water is not reported systematically; hence, the magnitude of this problem is essentially unknown. Fresh-water lakes and ocean beaches as well as swimming pools and whirlpool baths have all been implicated in the spread of disease. Infectious illnesses transmitted by recreational water use include folliculitis, otitis externa, diarrheal diseases, and such exotic infections as leptospirosis and primary amebic meningo-encephalitis. Increased rates of diarrheal illness among swimmers have been documented even at beaches where the water met EPA-recommended standards (Cabelli, Dufour, Levin, et al., 1979), suggesting that these standards may not be adequate.

Agents Responsible for Water-borne Disease

The specific etiology of about half of all water-borne disease outbreaks reported in the United States is never discovered. The remainder are caused by a handful of parasites, bacteria, viruses, and chemicals.

1. *Parasites.* A protozoan, *Giardia lamblia*, is responsible for more reported outbreaks of water-borne disease and more cases than any other organism. It was the cause of over half of such cases reported in 1981 (CDC, 1982), and in recent years has been implicated in a number of major municipal epidemics (Craun, 1979). Giardiasis, a nonfatal gastrointestinal illness, is characterized by intermittent diarrhea, bloating, and malabsorption. It is diagnosed by finding the organism in either its encysted or its motile (trophozoite) form on microscopic examination of the stool, but finding the organism may be difficult. The examination of numerous stools or even duodenal fluid may be required. For this reason, once the organism has been identified as responsible for an outbreak of illness, cases may be added to the total on the basis of symptoms alone, without laboratory confirmation. *Giardia* may enter a water supply as the result of fecal contamination either by humans or by wild animals, which are known to carry the parasite. *Giardia* cysts are not destroyed by ordinary water purification methods.

Major water-borne outbreaks of amebic dysentary caused by finding the organism in either its encysted or its motile (trophocently as the 1950s (Beck & Davies, 1981), but no such outbreaks have been reported in recent years. In this country, where the infection is uncommon, the usual route of transmission is person to person.

An estimated 200 million persons in Africa, Asia, and Latin America suffer from schistosomiasis (Hunter, Swartzwelder, & Clyde, 1976). Three species of *Schistosoma* parasites infect humans: *S. mansoni* (Africa and Latin America), *S. hematobium* (Africa), and *S. japonicum* (Asia). *S. hematobium* damages the bladder and may lead to bladder cancer; the other two species chiefly cause liver disease.

Humans become infected when wading or swimming in water that was contaminated previously with feces or urine containing schistosome eggs. The eggs release the free-swimming miracidial form of the parasite, which penetrates the host's skin. Aquatic snails serve as intermediate hosts; the disease is not transmitted in the United States because the requisite snail species do not live here.

Dracunculiasis (Guinea worm), a parasitic nematode infection found in India and Africa, is acquired by drinking contaminated water. A copepod—a tiny aquatic crustacean—serves as intermediate host and transmits the disease when ingested (Hunter et al., 1976). The worm lives in the subcutaneous tissues of the host; it often causes leg ulcers. An estimated 50 million people are infected.

2. *Bacteria*. *Salmonella* and *Shigella* have long been recognized as agents of water-borne illness in this country, and reports of outbreaks continue to occur on a yearly basis. Shigellosis, however, is more commonly transmitted person to person (Levine, 1981); and salmonellosis is usually a food-borne disease (Seals, 1981). Both salmonellosis and shigellosis are characterized by the acute onset of diarrhea, sometimes containing blood or mucus, and fever. Both infections are generally self-limited, although asymptomatic carriage of *Salmonella* may persist for months.

Salmonella typhi is the agent of typhoid fever, a disease that is now uncommon in this country. The most recent water-borne outbreak of this disease was reported in 1974 (Horwitz, Hughes, & Craun, 1976).

Cholera, caused by *Vibrio cholerae,* often is spread by contaminated water and has become a worldwide problem of pandemic proportions in recent years. Although totally absent from this country between 1911 and 1973, cholera has since reoccurred along the Gulf coast (Blake, Allegra, Snyder, et al., 1980). A 1978 outbreak of 11 cases in Louisiana was caused by eating inadequately cooked crabs, and a 1981 outbreak of 18 cases was caused by a contaminated water supply on a Texas oil rig (*Morbidity and Mortality Weekly Report,* 1981).

Enterotoxigenic *Escherichia coli* has long been suspected as a cause of some of the outbreaks of water-borne gastroenteritis for which no organism is identified. However, only one outbreak due to this pathogen has been documented—a major incident involving over 1000 people at Crater Lake National Park, Oregon, in 1975 (Rosenberg, Koplan, Wachsmuth, et al., 1977). *Campylobacter fetus* ssp. *jejuni* also has been identified as the cause of a single major water-borne outbreak of diarrheal disease, a 1978 Vermont episode affecting about 3000 people (Haley, Gunn, Hughes, et al., 1980). Both of these organisms are relatively difficult to identify in the laboratory; it is likely that they are the cause of other outbreaks in which their role is not detected.

    3.   *Viruses.* Among viral causes, water-borne transmission of hepatitis A is a well-known phenomenon, although, since 1974, only two water-borne outbreaks have been reported (CDC, 1982). In recent years, newer laboratory techniques have made it possible to identify the viruses responsible for some outbreaks of gastroenteritis; those implicated in water-borne illness to date have been parvovirus-like agents. Other viruses, such as rotavirus and enterovirus, are suspected of causing some water-borne outbreaks.

    4.   *Chemicals.* This is the final category of water-borne disease agents. Although not infectious, chemical outbreaks are included here because they are reported with outbreaks of water-borne infectious disease. A single case of an acute chemical intoxication that can be traced to drinking water is considered an outbreak. Agents most commonly implicated are heavy metals, usually from industrial sources, and fluoride from faulty fluoridation of drinking water. Between 1971 and 1978, 23 chemical outbreaks were reported (CDC, 1980).

FOOD-BORNE INFECTIOUS DISEASE

    Like water-borne disease, the great majority of acute illnesses transmitted by food are never reported; hence, the magnitude of this problem can only be estimated. In 1981, 568 outbreaks involving 14,432 cases were reported through public health agencies (CDC, 1983). These numbers are consistent with the 300 to 600 outbreaks, involving 10,000 to 20,000 people, which are reported each year (Black, Cox, & Horowitz, 1978). It is estimated, however, that as many as a million people yearly may be affected.

Contamination of Food

Any of several factors may be implicated in an episode or outbreak of food-borne illness (Bryan, 1978). These include:

1. *Improper holding temperatures.* Inadequate refrigeration is responsible for the majority of bacterial food-borne disease. Whether bacteria are introduced during food production or food handling, they require time, warmth, and moisture to multiply sufficiently for the food to become infective. Holding food at temperatures below 40° F will prevent the multiplication of most bacteria.

2. *Inadequate cooking.* This factor is responsible for many episodes of bacterial food-borne illness and most cases of food-borne parasitic disease. Food contaminated during production — such as *Salmonella*-contaminated meat — may be rendered safe by cooking sufficiently to bring all parts of the meat to a temperature above 160° F. Similarly, encysted larvae of parasites such as tapeworms and *Trichinella* may be destroyed by adequate cooking.

3. *Contaminated equipment.* Food grinders, meat slicers, cutting boards, and the like may be used to prepare contaminated food (i.e., raw meat) and subsequently employed, without proper cleaning, to prepare other foods, resulting in their contamination.

4. *Infected food handlers.* *Staphylococcus* and *Salmonella* bacteria and hepatitis virus, among others, are organisms that may be carried asymptomatically by food handlers. Proper personal hygiene — including hand washing — and heat-processing of foods after handling are protective measures.

5. *Food from unsafe sources.* Foods implicated in chemical outbreaks — such as toxic fish or mushrooms — are not contaminated by handling, nor can they generally be rendered safe in preparation. In these cases, the food itself is said to be unsafe.

Organisms Responsible for Food-borne Disease

The causes of the majority of food-borne outbreaks, like most water-borne outbreaks, are never defined. Of those for which an etiology is determined, about two-thirds are bacterial in origin, about one-sixth are chemical, and the remainder are viral or parasitic. The greatest number are caused by one of two bacteria: *Salmonella* and *Staphylococcus aureus*. There are over 200 other known causes of food-borne illness (Bryan, 1975); only a few can be discussed here.

1.   *Bacteria*. About 30 to 40 percent of bacterial food-borne outbreaks — about 25 percent of all food-borne outbreaks of known etiology — are caused by *Salmonella*. *Salmonella* food poisoning (like water-borne salmonellosis) is characterized by an incubation period of 18 to 24 hours and a clinical syndrome marked by fever, watery diarrhea that may contain blood or mucus, and vomiting. Symptoms usually subside within a few days, but the carrier state may persist for weeks or even months. *Salmonella typhi* is the etiologic agent of typhoid fever, a disease that is now uncommon in the United States.

Salmonella commonly infects domestic animals raised for food production, and current methods of processing and shipping foods in bulk makes this organism a frequent contaminant of meat. About 33 percent of poultry, 15 percent of pork, and up to 10 percent of beef products are contaminated with *Salmonella*. Eggs and animal products such as carmine dye also often are contaminated. The organism is destroyed by cooking but may survive temperatures less than 160° F. This creates problems for persons who like their roast beef rare, and for commercial food preparers. *Salmonella* may be passed on to other foods by utensils, surfaces, or personnel used in preparing raw meat. Other sources of *Salmonella* in the environment include pets such as baby chicks or turtles.

Staphylococcus aureus is the cause of about one-quarter of all bacterial food-borne outbreaks. Food-borne infection with this organism usually results in a gastrointestinal syndrome with vomiting following an incubation period of two to four hours. The illness is self-limited, with symptoms usually subsiding in a few hours.

Staphylococcus aureus is most commonly introduced into food by handlers, who may carry the organism, without symptoms, in the nose or throat. If the food is not adequately refrigerated, the bacteria will multiply, producing a toxin; it is this toxin that is responsible for the illness caused by contaminated food. The toxin is heat-stable and so is not destroyed by cooking.

Clostridium botulinum is the causative agent of botulism, a potentially fatal illness characterized by cranial nerve palsies followed by paralysis of the extremities and the muscles of respiration. The organism is anaerobic and spore-forming; the spores germinate and the bacteria produce toxin under conditions of low oxygen tension, such as in improperly canned food. The toxin is heat-labile, so it may be destroyed by cooking. Because of its severity, virtually all outbreaks of botulism are reported to public health authorities; an average of about 15 per year are reported in the United States (CDC, 1983).

Other bacteria reported with some frequency in food-borne outbreaks are *Clostridium perfringens; Shigella;* and *Vibrio parahemolyticus.* All of these produce diarrheal disease. An additional 15 species of bacteria were identified rarely as the cause of food-borne outbreaks between 1977 and 1981 (CDC, 1983).

2. *Viruses.* Although viral gastroenteritis may be transmitted by food, reports of such transmission are quite rare. Non-B hepatitis is the only viral illness commonly identified in food-borne outbreaks; 30 such outbreaks were reported between 1977 and 1981 (CDC, 1983). Hepatitis virus may be introduced into food by asymptomatic carriers serving as food handlers.

3. *Parasites: Trichinella spiralis* is the most common food-borne parasite in the United States; it is transmitted through undercooked pork or, occasionally, bear meat. Since the practice of feeding uncooked garbage to hogs generally has been abandoned in recent years, trichinosis has become less common; since 1963, fewer than 200 cases per year have been reported (CDC, 1981).

Beef, pork, and fish tapeworms, transmitted through the undercooked flesh of the intermediate host, are occasionally acquired in the United States; and *Giardia lamblia* (which is usually water-borne) and *Entameba histolytica* (which is usually transmitted person to person) sometimes may be food-borne. Flukes, such as *Clonorchis sinensis,* are transmitted in the far east through the consumption of raw crustaceans and occasionally may be found in the United States in immigrants.

4. *Chemicals.* Although not infectious, chemical outbreaks are included here because they are reported together with food-borne outbreaks of infectious disease and account for 20 to 25 percent of all food-borne outbreaks of known etiology reported annually in the United States. Poisoning with scombrotoxin and ciguatoxin are reported most frequently; these are naturally produced toxins occurring in certain types of fish. Scombrotoxin is associated with fish such as amberjack, red snapper, grouper, and barracuda, while ciguatoxin is found most often in a Hawaiian dish known as mahi-mahi. Scombrotoxin generally causes flushing, headache, and allergic symptoms; ciguatoxin poisoning results in paresthesias (tingling sensations of the mouth and extremities). Twenty to 40 such outbreaks per year are reported (CDC, 1983).

Acute outbreaks of food-borne poisoning due to heavy metals, mushrooms, paralytic shellfish toxins (caused by "red tides" affecting shellfish beds), and other chemicals are reported in small numbers each year.

VECTOR-BORNE INFECTIOUS DISEASE

The term "vector" denotes a nonhuman carrier of disease organisms that can transmit these organisms directly to humans. The term implies that an active role is played by the carrier; if the carrier is ingested by humans, it is considered an intermediate host (e.g., the role of swine in trichinosis). Usually the term refers to insects or rodents.

Vectors may be either biological or mechanical. In the former, the pathogenic microorganism must multiply or develop within the vector before becoming infective. The time required to do so is the *extrinsic incubation period* of the disease. Mechanical vectors, on the other hand, simply transport microorganisms from one place to another; houseflies and cockroaches are examples.

As is true in the case of most infectious disease, vector-borne illness is of much greater importance in the developing world than in industrialized countries. Malaria, transmitted by mosquitoes, is perhaps the most widespread, serious disease among humans. Other insect-borne diseases that are unknown in the United States, such as yellow fever, filariasis, and kala-azar, cause considerable suffering and death in much of the world.

Insect Vectors

Mosquitoes.   As shown in Table 2–2, mosquitoes are responsible for the transmission of a variety of pathogenic organisms, including viruses, protozoa, and metazoa. The importance of mos-

Table 2-2   Some Insect Vectors and Diseases Transmitted by Them

Vector	Disease	Pathogen
Mosquitoes		
Anopheles sp.	Malaria	*Plasmodium sp.* (protozoa)
Culex sp.	Filiariasis	*Wucheraria bancrofti* and *malayi* (nematodes)
Culex sp.	Encephalitis	arbovirus
Aedes aegypti	Yellow fever	arbovirus
Aedes aegypti	Dengue	arbovirus
Biting Flies		
Deerfly	Filariasis	*Loa loa* (nematode)
Black fly	River blindness	*Onchocerca volvulus* (nematode)
Tsetse fly	Sleeping sickness	*Trypanosoma gambiense* and *rhodesiense* (protozoa)
Sand fly	Kala-azar	*Leishmania donovani*
	Tropical ulcer	*Leishmania tropica*
	Cutaneous leishmaniasis	*Leishmania mexicana*
	Espundia	*Leishmania braziliense* (protozoa)
	Phlebotomus fever	arbovirus
Other Insects		
Gnats	Filariasis	*Mansonella ozzardi* (nematode)
Rat flea	Plague	*Yersinia pestis* (bacteria)
	Murine typhus	*Rickettsia mooseri*
Body louse	Epidemic typhus	*Rickettsia prowazekii*
	Trench fever	*Rickettsia quintana*
Tick	Rocky Mountain spotted fever	*Rickettsia rickettsia*
Tick	Colorado tick fever	arbovirus
Mite	Rickettsialpox	*Rickettsia akari*

quitoes as vectors of disease, as well as their nuisance value, has led to widespread efforts to control them. The mosquito-control specialist must have a thorough knowledge of mosquito habits and ecology. All mosquitoes breed in stagnant water and produce aquatic larvae, but the type of water (polluted pond, salt marsh, etc.) preferred by different species varies. Some species of mosquitoes may fly up to 20 miles, while the effective range of *Aedes aegypti* is limited to about one block (Savage, 1980).

Mosquito surveillance is conducted to gain information regarding changes in the numbers and varieties of mosquitoes present in an area where control operations are to be conducted. A variety of traps is used to collect adults; larvae are dipped manually from collections of stagnant water. In malarious areas, adult mosquitoes may be dissected and their stomachs and salivary glands examined microscopically to determine the rate of carriage of malaria parasites (Hunter et al., 1976, p. 379).

There are three fundamental types of mosquito control: environmental, chemical, and biological.

1. *Environmental control.* The elimination of mosquito breeding sites and the use of screening and/or bed nets are the oldest of mosquito control methods. Methods such as these were the chief tools in celebrated campaigns such as those of Major William Gorgas to eliminate yellow fever from Havana and the Panama Canal Zone in the early 1900s. Application of environmental control measures includes the elimination of human-made breeding sites, such as collections of water in tin cans, flower pots, discarded tires, and other refuse; the use of proper irrigation practices; and the modification or filling of natural breeding sites such as marshes.

2. *Chemical control.* Since World War II, a great number of insecticides, both larvacides and adulticides, have become available. These generally are classified as stomach poisons, which must be ingested; contact poisons, which penetrate the insect's cuticle; or fumigants, which are inhaled by the insect through its spiracles (Pratt, Littig, & Barnes, 1960).

Insecticides have been used widely throughout the world in programs for the control of malaria and other vector-borne illnesses, and to these chemicals have been attributed a large share of whatever success the programs have attained. In recent years, however, two major problems have emerged in the use of insecticides. First is the problem of insect resistance to these chemicals. Over 200 species of insects have developed resistance to one or more insecticides, and compounds such as DDT, which were once the mainstay of most mosquito-control programs in tropical areas, have now become almost useless in many places (Beck & Davies, 1981).

The other problem is increasing recognition of the potential dangers to the health of humans and other higher animals that may be posed by the insecticides themselves. Acute poisoning incidents have always been a well-known threat, but the possible long-term consequences of insecticide exposure only recently have become a matter for concern. DDT, for instance, is known to be concentrated through the food chain, stored in fat, and secreted in human milk (Woodard, Ferguson, & Wilson, 1976). It is known to cause weakening of the shells of eggs laid by exposed birds, but its effects in humans are still a matter of speculation. Considerations such as these have led to the elimination of the use of DDT in the United States and the heavy regulation of the use of other insecticides (see Chapters 3 and 8). Ultralow volume techniques — in which small amounts of insecticide are spread over a wide area by airplane — have come into use as a method for reducing the dangers of human exposure.

3. *Biological control.* A variety of biological methods — including the use of pheromones, microorganisms, and sterilized males — have been used to control various insect pests. Only one such method so far has been found to have utility in mosquito control: the stocking of permanent bodies of water with small fish (*Gambusia*) that feed on mosquito larvae.

There are several diseases transmitted by mosquitoes (see Table 2-2):

1. *Malaria.* Malaria is endemic throughout most of the non-industrialized world. Until about 1975, it appeared that programs of mosquito control and treatment of cases were bringing this disease generally under control. More recently, however, it has become apparent that its prevalence is increasing. Worldwide, it is estimated that over 200 million people (almost equivalent to the U.S. population) are infected.

Until the early 1950s, malaria was endemic in the southeastern United States. Importation of cases to this country continues to occur: A peak number of 4247 imported cases was recorded in 1970 (during the Vietnam War); in 1982, 930 cases were imported (CDC, 1984). Despite the presence of anophelene mosquitoes, however, transmission of malaria occurs only rarely in the United States. This is apparently because a *critical density* of anophelene mosquitoes and infected persons is required to sustain transmission (Plorde, 1977); therefore, a relatively few imported cases do not constitute a sufficient parasite reservoir.

Malaria is caused by a protozoan parasite that reproduces within the host's red blood cells. It is characterized by periodic chills and fever; adult hosts in endemic areas may possess a high degree of acquired immunity and be relatively asymptomatic for long periods of time. Four species of the *Plasmodium* genus are responsible for human malaria: *P. vivax,* the most common, causes tertian malaria (a three-day fever cycle); *P. malariae* causes quartan malaria (a four-day fever cycle); *P. falciparum* causes malignant tertian malaria, the most serious form of the disease; and *P. ovale* causes ovale tertian malaria, a relatively mild illness.

2.   *Yellow Fever.* This is caused by an arbovirus and is found in South America and Africa. The virus attacks the liver, kidneys, and brain, and the illness is marked by jaundice and hemorrhage.

Epidemics of yellow fever in the United States occurred as far north as New York in the eighteenth century. It was not until the early 1900s — following the pioneering work of Walter Reed and Carlos Findlay in identifying the mosquito vector — that the disease was eliminated from New Orleans (Williams, 1959).

Yellow fever occurs in two cycles: urban and jungle (or sylvatic). Jungle yellow fever is maintained in a mosquito–monkey cycle and is transmitted by several species of mosquito that breed and dwell in the jungle canopy. If a human is bitten by one of these vectors — as sometimes happens in clearing jungle land for farming or road building — the person may contract the disease and return to the city to initiate the urban, human–*Aedes aegypti* cycle.

3.   *Other arboviruses.* Numerous arboviruses cause disease in humans; few of these are found in the United States. Most are transmitted by mosquitoes; some are spread by ticks. Arbovirus infections are marked by fever, headache, and myalgia; some include hemorrhagic phenomena, central nervous system involvement, and other symptoms.

Several types of arboviral encephalitis are transmitted in the United States; these include Eastern equine, Western equine, and St. Louis encephalitis. None are common, although occasional outbreaks occur.

Dengue is an illness characterized by aching and fever. It

is fairly common in the Caribbean and elsewhere in the tropics; in 1980, the first U.S. cases since 1945 were reported in Texas (*Morbidity and Mortality Weekly Report,* 1980).

Flies.   As with mosquitoes, a knowledge of fly ecology is important to the control of these insects. The breeding patterns and flight ranges of different species vary widely. Fly traps and other devices are available as aids in surveillance.

Control of domestic flies is attained best through proper disposal of wastes. The use of screens is important; insecticides usually are used in a variety of baits and strips. Flies often are resistant to many insecticides (Savage, 1980).

The control of sylvatic biting flies, which serve as biological vectors of disease, often is difficult. Blackflies (*Simulium*), for instance, which transmit river blindness (onchocerciasis), breed only in fast-flowing water. Attempts to control this insect have involved the aerial larvaciding of hard-to-reach rapids in west Africa.

As shown in Table 2-2, a number of diseases are transmitted by biting flies. In the United States, however, biting flies are not significant carriers of disease. Occasionally, they may serve as mechanical vectors of tularemia or anthrax (American Academy of Pediatrics, 1982), but the former is uncommon (150 to 250 cases/yr) and the latter is essentially nonexistent in this country. Biting flies such as black flies and horseflies may be significant nuisances.

In tropical countries, on the other hand, biting flies are important vectors of parasitic disease, as shown in Table 2-2. In some areas, these exotic diseases are of great importance: Onchocerciasis is a major cause of blindness in parts of western Africa; while sleeping sickness, which affects both humans and cattle, makes substantial tracts of otherwise arable land in Africa virtually uninhabitable.

Diseases also are transmitted by domestic flies. Houseflies breed in excrement, garbage, and other waste and have been implicated as mechanical vectors in the spread of typhoid fever, bacterial diarrheas, amebiasis, trachoma, and other diseases (Benenson, 1980). Their relative importance in the spread of infectious disease, however, is largely unknown.

Any of several species of fly may be responsible for myiasis, a condition in which eggs are deposited in a wound and fly larvae subsequently invade the surrounding tissue.

Other Insect Vectors. As shown in Table 2–2, a variety of other biting insects serve as biological vectors for a number of illnesses, including those caused by parasites, bacteria, viruses, and *Rickettsia*. In the United States, the most important of these is Rocky Mountain spotted fever, transmitted by the bite of ticks of the genus *Dermacentor*. It is actually most prevalent in the Appalachian Mountain states and occurs relatively infrequently in the Rockies. Hikers, hunters, and backpackers are at particular risk. Approximately 1000 cases are reported annually in the United States.

Plague, well known for the devastation it caused in Europe in the Middle Ages, occurs occasionally (5 to 10 cases/yr) in the western United States, where rodents such as prairie dogs serve as reservoirs. Human cases occur chiefly in persons engaged in outdoor work or recreation.

Filariasis is an infection caused by several species of roundworm and it is found in Africa, Asia, and the Pacific; as shown in Table 2–2, it has several vectors. It is characterized by subcutaneous nodules, recurring fevers, and, with some species of parasite, lymphedema of the lower extremities and scrotum.

Other diseases for which insects serve as specific vectors are either rare (murine typhus, Colorado tick fever) or nonexistent in the United States. Some biting insects such as head lice and bedbugs are nuisances but do not transmit any disease.

Common household insects such as cockroaches have been shown to carry pathogenic organisms and are thought to serve as mechanical vectors of diarrheal and other diseases. Their actual role in disease transmission, however, remains largely undefined.

Rodent Vectors

Domestic rats and mice are highly adaptable creatures; they live in both urban and rural areas, in and around the various structures built by humans. Surveillance is conducted chiefly by experienced inspectors searching for droppings, runways, and other signs of rodent presence.

Control efforts are based on both environmental and chemical methods. The former are preferred; they involve making dwellings and food as inaccessible as possible to rodents. Buildings are "rat-proofed" by sealing holes around plumbing, under doors, and so on. Leaks in sewers are repaired; refuse is disposed of properly.

Several rodenticides are used in rat control, mostly mixed with baits. During the last 10 years, strains of rats resistant to some of these poisons — particularly the anticoagulants, such as Warfarin — have emerged (Savage, 1980).

As carriers of disease, two species of rat are of public health importance: the Norway rat (*Rattus norvegicus*) and the roof rat (*Rattus rattus*). These animals may serve as reservoir hosts or biological or mechanical vectors of disease. In addition, the house mouse (*Mus musculus*) may serve as a reservoir host or mechanical vector (Savage, 1980).

Rats serve as reservoirs of plague and murine typhus, diseases which are transmitted by the rat flea. They also are reservoirs of trichinosis. The house mouse is a reservoir for rickettsialpox, a rare illness that is transmitted by a mite that parasitizes the mouse.

Rats and mice are thought to serve as mechanical vectors of salmonellosis; they carry the organisms in their intestines and may contaminate human food with their droppings. Rats also serve as mechanical vectors and reservoirs for leptospirosis, as do many other domestic and wild animals. Leptospirosis, a flulike illness that sometimes includes hemorrhage and jaundice, is caused by a bacterium, *Leptospira icterohemorrhagiae*. Humans usually contract the disease when swimming or working in water contaminated with animal urine; the bacteria enter through an open cut or sore (Benenson, 1980).

Rats are biological vectors for rat-bite fever, a rare but occasionally fatal febrile illness caused by the bacteria *Streptobaccilus moniliformis* or *Spirillum minus*. Rat bites themselves are much more common than most of the infectious diseases carried by rats, particularly in depressed urban areas. Children are often the victims. In the third world, one of the greatest problems posed by rats is their consumption of stored foodstuffs.

SOIL-BORNE PARASITIC DISEASE

Soil-borne parasites are among the most common infectious diseases in the world. It is estimated that one-quarter of the world's population (650 million people) is infected with the large roundworm, *Ascaris lumbricoides,* and about 450 million persons are infected with hookworm (Beck & Davies, 1981).

In the United States, these infections are limited chiefly to the rural southeastern states. While not as prevalent as in years past, there remain communities where 50 percent or more of the children are infected with *Ascaris* (Schultz, 1974). It is estimated that in this country, 4 million persons are infected with *Ascaris*; 2.2 million with whipworm; 700,000 with hookworm; and 400,000 with *Strongyloides stercoralis* (Warren, 1972).

These parasites are dependent for their transmission on human feces being deposited on the ground; the eggs or larvae undergo a period of development in the soil. They are therefore prevalent in association with rural poverty and its attendant conditions of poor sanitation and education.

Proper disposal of human feces is central to the control of these parasites. Construction of privies may be helpful. Periodic mass treatment of children in communities where *Ascaris* is prevalent provides at least temporary control of this parasite. The wearing of shoes protects against hookworm and *Strongyloides*. However, soil-borne nematodes are likely to remain common where rural poverty is present and soil and climatic conditions permit. Control of the parasites ultimately will depend on the elimination of this poverty.

The following are the more common soil-borne parasitic diseases.

1. *Ascaris.* Roundworm ova are ingested by the host and hatch in the small intestine. The larvae then undertake a bizarre migration through the body of the host: They penetrate the intestinal wall, enter the venous circulation, and are filtered out in the lungs. As they migrate through the lungs, they may cause a type of pneumonia (Loeffler's syndrome). The larvae then ascend the bronchi and trachea, are swallowed, and return to the small intestine, where they mature, mate, and produce eggs. A single female *Ascaris* can produce 200,000 eggs per day.

A host may harbor hundreds of worms, and a bolus of worms may cause intestinal obstruction, a complication that is not rare in areas of high prevalence in the southeastern United States. Other complications generally are seen only in the tropics: A worm may perforate the intestine, obstruct the common bile or pancreatic duct, or cause appendicitis, intussception, or volvulus. In addition, a heavy infection may have an adverse nutritional effect on the host.

2. *Hookworm*. This parasite was once very common in the southeastern United States and was responsible for widespread serious morbidity. The work of the Rockefeller Sanitary Commission from 1910 to 1920 was responsible for a great reduction in its prevalence, and it has continued to decline since.

Hookworm ova hatch in the soil and the larvae enter the host's body by penetrating the skin – usually through bare feet. They then undertake a migration identical to that of *Ascaris* larvae. In the small intestine, the adults attach themselves to the intestinal mucosa and actively suck blood. A heavy infection ("hookworm disease") can cause severe anemia, hypoproteinemia, edema, and congestive heart failure.

3. *Whipworm*. These parasites enter the host's body when the ova are ingested. The larvae pass directly to the large intestine, where they mature and can cause diarrhea. A heavy infection can result in rectal prolapse.

4. *Strongyloides*. The *Strongyloides* ova hatch in the intestine of the host, and larvae are passed in the stool. The larvae may enter a free-living cycle in the soil or may invade the body of a new host through the skin and migrate as do hookworm larvae. Larvae in the host intestine also may penetrate directly through the intestinal mucosa to establish a new migratory cycle, a process known as internal autoinfection. *Strongyloides* is particularly dangerous to the malnourished or immunocompromised host: Massive internal auto-infection takes place, larvae migrate aberrantly throughout the body (the "hyperinfection syndrome"), and shock and death may result.

5. *Animal nematodes*. The larvae of dog or cat hookworms may penetrate the skin of a human, but their migration is limited to the skin. A highly pruritic rash, known as cutaneous larva migrans or "creeping eruption," results. This condition is encountered not uncommonly in bathers on beaches where dogs run loose.

If the ova of dog or cat ascarids (*Toxocara canis* and *Toxocara cati*) are ingested by a human, the larvae migrate aberrantly and enter the liver, the eye, or even the brain – a disease known as visceral larva migrans. The condition is most common in the children of dog owners (Schantz, Weiss, Pollard, & White, 1980).

REFERENCES

American Academy of Pediatrics (1982). *Report of the Committee on Infectious Diseases,* 19th ed. Evanston, Ill.: AAP.

Beck, J. W., and Davies, J. E. (1981). *Medical Parasitology,* 3rd ed. St. Louis: C. V. Mosby.

Benenson, A. (ed.) (1980). *Control of Communicable Disease in Man,* 13th ed. Washington, D.C.: American Public Health Association.

Black, R. E., Cox, R. C., and Horwitz, M. A. (1978). Outbreaks of Food-borne Disease in the United States, 1975. *J Infectious Dis* 137:213–218.

Blake, P. A., Allegra, D. T., Snyder, J. D., et al. (1980). Cholera—A Possible Endemic Focus in the United States. *New Eng J Med* 302:305–309.

Bryan, F. A. (1975). *Disease Transmitted by Foods.* Atlanta: DHEW Publication No. (CDC) 75-8237.

Bryan, F. A. (1978). Factors That Contribute to Outbreaks of Food-borne Disease. *J Food Protection* 41:816–827.

Cabelli, V. J., Dufour, A. P., Levin, M. A., McCabe, L. J., and Haberman, P. W. (1979). Relationship of Microbial Indicators to Health Effects at Marine Bathing Beaches. *Am J Pub Health* 69:690–696.

Centers for Disease Control (1980). *Water-related Disease Surveillance, Annual Summary, 1978.* Atlanta: USDHHS Publication No. (CDC) 80-8385.

Centers for Disease Control (1981). *Trichinosis Surveillance, Annual Summary, 1980.* Atlanta: USDHHS Publication No. (CDC) 81-8256.

Centers for Disease Control (1984). *Malaria Surveillance, Annual Summary, 1982.* Atlanta: USDHHS Publication.

Centers for Disease Control (1982). *Water-related Disease Outbreaks Surveillance, Annual Summary, 1981.* Atlanta: USDHHS Publication No. (CDC) 82-8385.

Centers for Disease Control (1983). *Food-borne Disease Surveillance, Annual Summary, 1981.* Atlanta: USDHHS Publication No. (CDC) 83-8185.

Craun, G. F. (1979). Water-borne Giardiasis in the United States: A Review. *Am J Pub Health* 69:817–819.

Haley, C. E., Gunn, R. A., Hughes, J. M., Lippy, E. C., and Craun, G. F. (1980). Outbreaks of Water-borne Disease in the United States, 1978. *J Infec Dis* 141:794–797.

Horwitz, M. A., Hughes, J. M., and Craun, G. F. (1976). Outbreaks of Water-borne Disease in the United States, 1974. *J Infec Dis* 133:588–593.

Hunter, G. W., Swartzwelder, J. C., and Clyde, D. F. (1976). *Tropical Medicine,* 5th ed. New York: W. B. Saunders.

Levine, M. M. (1981). Shigellosis. In P. F. Wehrle and F. H. Top (eds.), *Communicable and Infectious Diseases.* 9th ed. St. Louis: C. V. Mosby.

McGauhey, P. H. (1968). *Engineering Management of Water Quality.* New York: McGraw-Hill.

Morbidity and Mortality Weekly Report (1980). Dengue—United States. 29:531–532.

Morbidity and Mortality Weekly Report (1981). Cholera on a Gulf Coast Oil Rig—Texas. 30:589–590.

Plorde, J. J. (1977). Malaria. In Thorne, G. W., Adams, R. D., and Braunwald, E., *Harrison's Principles of International Medicine.* New York: McGraw-Hill.

Pratt, H. D., Littig, K. W., and Barnes, R. C. (1960). *Survey and Control of Mosquitoes of Public Health Importance.* Atlanta: USDHEW Publication No. VC-36.

Rosenberg, M. L., Koplan, J. P., Wachsmuth, I. K., et al. (1977). Epidemic Diarrhea at Crater Lake from Enterotoxigenic *Escherichia coli. Ann Intern Med* 86:714–718.

Savage, E. P. (1980). Disease Vectors. In P. W. Purdom, *Environmental Health.* New York: Academic Press.

Schantz, P. M., Weis, P. E., Pollard, Z. F., and White, M. C. (1980). Risk Factors for Toxocaral Ocular Larva Migrans: A Case-control Study. *Am J Pub Health* 70:1273–1277.

Schultz, M. G. (1974). The Surveillance of Parasitic Diseases in the United States. *Am J Trop Med Hyg* 23:744–751.

Seals, J. E. (1981). Nontyphoidal salmonellosis. In P. F. Wehrle and F. H. Top (eds.), *Communicable and Infectious Diseases,* 9th ed. St. Louis: C. V. Mosby.

Snow, J. (1855). *On the Mode of Communication of Cholera,* 2nd ed. London: Churchill. Quoted in Mausner, J. S., and Bahn, A. K. (1974). *Epidemiology: An Introductory Text.* Philadelphia: W. B. Saunders.

United States Environmental Protection Agency (1976). *Quality Criteria for Water.* Washington, D.C.: EPA.

Warren, K. S. (1972). Helminthic Diseases Endemic in the United States. *Am J Trop Med Hyg* 23:723–730.

Williams, G. (1959). *Virus Hunters.* New York: Alfred A. Knopf.

Woodard, B. T., Ferguson, B. B., and Wilson, D. J. (1976). DDT Levels in Milk of Rural Indigent Blacks. *Am J Dis Child* 130:400–403.

Chapter 3

Chemicals, Health, and the Environment

D. Peter Drotman *

It is very tempting to begin the chapter on chemicals in the environment by reviewing the dramatic environmental tragedies of the recent past such as Times Beach, Missouri; Love Canal in New York; the explosion of the Hoffmann-LaRoche subsidiary chemical plant in Seveso, Italy; the contamination with polybrominated biphenyls of virtually every milk consumer in Michigan due to an error in preparing cattle feed; the poignant and tragic story of Minamata Bay, Japan, where so many suffered irreversible neurologic disease after consuming fish contaminated with mercury wastes dumped into the water by local paper mills; along with many others.

Fascinating and important though these incidents are, they represent only the tip of the iceberg. Far more of the overall problem of chemicals in the environment is submerged and difficult to see. Only where large numbers of people are heavily exposed to an agent or agents have the incidents come to general attention and, all too often, only to the attention of medical, public health, and environmental professionals. However, even though there are significant scientific, medical, environmental, social, economic, and even ethical

---

*This chapter was written by Dr. Drotman in his private capacity. No official support or endorsement by the Centers for Disease Control or the Department of Health and Human Services is intended or should be inferred.

lessons to be learned from each of the environmental disasters just listed (and many others), the important issues of environmental health also concern the relatively low levels of agents to which virtually everyone on the planet is exposed on virtually a continual basis. The agents are as variable as the potential routes of exposure.

THE CHEMICAL CONTROVERSY: HOW MUCH IS HARMFUL?

As Paracelsus, the sixteenth-century Swiss physician who introduced lead and arsenic into pharmaceutical chemistry, indicated, only the dose of a substance determines its toxicity. In a pure sense, this is begging the question; excessive exposure to anything is bound to produce untoward effect. This notion leads to the controversy concerning the definition of hazardous environmental exposure to chemicals. In some ways, this is analogous to the problems we have with defining hazardous exposures to radiation. There is no doubt that large doses of radiation are harmful and possibly fatal. As will be discussed in Chapter 4, the controversy occurs at the other end of the dose/response curve. No one knows for sure what, if any, are the health effects to humans of small doses of radiation. Is the relationship between radiation dose and health effects linear; that is, do all doses above zero have some untoward effect in some people? Or is there a threshold, a level below which there is no harmful effect and above which such effects begin to occur?

So run the arguments surrounding chemicals, although chemicals are more complex and difficult to measure. Since everything that exists is made of chemicals, defining exposure to toxic chemicals is difficult, to say the least. Indeed, some chemicals are essential nutrients in small amounts but extremely toxic in slightly larger amounts. Examples of this would be copper, chromium, and possibly arsenic. These are needed to produce several enzymes but in larger doses can produce characteristic illnesses and even death. The beneficial aspect of many chemicals stands in contrast to radiation. Radiation is presumably beneficial when used in medicine and industry, but in general it is destructive to human health.

Humans have been exposed to some toxic chemicals, such as lead, from time immemorial (Ericson, Shirahata, & Patterson, 1979).

The health effects of exposures to low doses of lead (for instance, the amount absorbed into crops from soil and entered in the food chain), are controversial. Lead is toxic to the nervous and other organ systems. Some researchers have claimed that even minute exposures to lead are associated with behavior disorders in children (Needleman, Gunnoe, & Leviton, 1979). The use of lead in industry has increased exponentially for more than 200 years (Meadows, Meadows, Randers, & Behrens, 1974). Much of this lead has been discharged into the environment, as, for instance, in automobile exhaust. Studies of deep samples of the Greenland ice cap show that lead concentration in the hundreds-of-years-old layers of snow correlates with the age of the ice. Clearly, the increasing use of lead has resulted in the pollution of our entire planet with this metal.

There are other chemicals that have existed for only a short time, compared to the natural elements such as lead and mercury. The new synthetic compounds are products of the relatively young sciences of organic chemistry, physical chemistry, and biochemistry. The best known of these compounds are DDT and polychlorinated biphenyls (PCBs). Chlorinated aromatic hydrocarbons such as these were first synthesized about 100 years ago. Both DDT and PCBs have become environmental disaster stories that rival, and probably exceed, in their significance the environmental dispersion of fallout from nuclear weapons testing.

Although DDT was first synthesized in 1874, it was not until 1936 that Paul Miller discovered it to be insecticidal. This observation brought him a Nobel prize in 1948. Extensive use of DDT was delayed by World War II, but, once begun, countless tons were used all over the world (Davies & Edmundson, 1972).

DDT was seen as a saving grace for humanity. Its insecticidal properties could be used to increase food and fiber crop yields by decreasing losses to insects. There was hope that DDT use could eventuate in the eradication of malaria and other mosquito and insect-borne diseases. This was considered particularly beneficial because malaria was responsible for more deaths than any other disease in the world. At first, DDT appeared to live up to its promise but, as described later in this chapter, it later seemed to turn on its creators. It is now banned in the United States and many other nations and is used much less than in the past in other countries.

The saga of PCBs is similar but somewhat less well known.

PCBs are semisynthetic, chlorinated hydrocarbon oils used extensively since about 1930. PCBs are virtually indestructible. They do not burn or react readily. They also have dielectric properties that make them very useful in the electric-power and electronics industries as transformer and capacitor fluids. They are so good for this purpose that virtually every one of the millions of capacitors and transformers manufactured in this country between the 1930s and 1970s contained PCBs in volumes ranging from a few milliliters to hundreds of liters.

It is ironic that the very properties that made PCBs useful made them environmental and, in some instances, public health disasters. The chemical inertness and stability that made them useful as electrical insulators and coolants translated into nondegradability and bioaccumulation once they came to be released into the environment. PCBs began to be phased out by Monsanto, the only company that manufactured them in this country, in the early 1970s. By the end of the 1970s, manufacture and all new uses ceased. However, tons of PCBs remain in use. Since the useful life of the equipment that contains PCBs is many years, the threat of continued environmental contamination with PCBs is a real one (Schneider, 1979).

How and why these and other chemicals came to be environmental threats instead of economic boons is a central message of this chapter. How humans came to be exposed to these and other chemicals is another important theme. Listing all the possible health effects of various chemicals, however, is well beyond the scope of this book. Indeed, considerable biomedical research continues to be concentrated in just this area. Our knowledge of environmental chemicals evolves rapidly and is revised nearly as rapidly. Knowing sources of data and information is the key to being scientifically accurate in environmental matters. Therefore, this chapter will include pointers on where to seek timely data and current expertise on chemicals and health effects of chemicals.

HISTORICAL REVIEW: CHEMICALS IN SOCIAL CONTEXT

As has been discussed elsewhere in this and other community medicine and public health texts, health problems and concerns do not exist in a vacuum. They are logical derivations of human activity and natural conditions (Read, 1966). As social and scientific change take place, so do health problems change. The development of specific jobs can mean different milieus and exposures for different groups. For example, Rome was one of the first societies to have a piped water supply. The pipes were fashioned from lead, a metal that is pliant yet sufficiently durable for this purpose. The Latin word for lead is "plumbum." This root word gives us the chemical symbol for lead, Pb, as well as the name of the vocation concerned with water pipes — plumber.

Lead is a toxic substance. It is particularly toxic to the nervous system, and children are especially susceptible to its effects. If lead is drunk, even in tiny amounts dissolved in drinking water, it is well-absorbed from the gastrointestinal tract and deposited in the central nervous system. When a sufficient amount accumulates, lead encephalopathy may be a severe result. Some historians have theorized that this may explain the fall of the Roman Empire (Mack, 1973; Waldron, 1973). Obviously, only the upper-class citizens of Rome would have had water piped into their homes. According to the theory, their children drank the water and were exposed to the lead, putting them at high risk for lead neurotoxicity. Since so many of these children were unable to reach their full mental potential, and since the upper class ruled Rome, there developed a scarcity of leadership for the society. Lead toxicity also may explain some of the bizarre behavior of some of the notorious Roman Emperors.

As people came together to live in cities, health problems changed yet again. Crowded conditions meant that infections transmitted from person to person (such as smallpox) and those borne by vectors (such as plague) could occur in great epidemics. It is estimated that one of every three persons in Europe died of plague during the great epidemics of the fourteenth century.

Industries grew and hence so did the use of metals, minerals, oils, and solvents. Sir Percival Pott in 1775 was the first to describe an environmental carcinogen (Kipling & Waldron, 1976). He found cancer of the scrotum among young boys who worked as chimney sweeps in London in the latter half of the eighteenth century. Soot collected in the rugae of the boys' scrotums and resulted in the cancer. However, it was not until this century that the specific component of the soot that caused the cancer was identified. The polycyclic aromatic hydrocarbon, benzo (a) pyrene is found naturally in coal, petroleum, tar, and some wood. Although social changes that preclude child labor have halted the types of exposure Pott discovered, benzo (a) pyrene is a constituent of air pollution (from combustion of gasoline). Many coal, petroleum, and shale oil workers continue to be exposed to this carcinogen on their jobs. It is also a component of tobacco smoke.

PETROLEUM, PETROCHEMICALS, AND THE ENVIRONMENT

The petroleum industry has been a paradigm of American "progress"; and, indeed, we owe this industry a great debt for what the United States is today—both good and bad. Because the growth of this industry teaches us so much about what we are—not only chemically but socially, economically, and in many other ways—it is worthwhile learning more about it.

Petroleum and petrochemicals play a greater role in our lives than we generally realize. Beyond the obvious uses of petroleum as fuel for our cars and electrical power plants, petroleum-derived compounds make up most of the plastics, pesticides, and fertilizers we use; most of our synthetic fiber garments; and many of the medicines we use and prescribe daily, including isopropyl alcohol. In this chapter we are concerned only with the environmental and health impacts of petroleum and its many derivatives; thus, we will not discuss the political and economic aspects of this natural resource.

Petroleum has been used virtually throughout history. It was accessible historically via natural surface seepage sites, and its chief uses were as fuel (kerosene) and pitch (tar for sealing vessels). Petroleum nowadays is taken from deep underground by highly sophisticated drilling processes. It emerges from the ground as crude oil and is refined into a number of fractions. The lightest fractions, containing very short-chain alkyl compounds, are combined to form longer-chain compounds. This light fraction is used to manufacture gasoline, which in its final form is a mixture of several hundred compounds. The demand for gasoline, beginning at the end of the nineteenth century, grew coincident with the popularity of vehicles powered by internal combustion engines.

When World War I began in 1914, there was an abrupt need for acetone, a basic material for the manufacture of explosives. Until then, most acetone was derived from isopropyl alcohol, the source of which was wood distillation. After the war, the new process of thermal cracking of petroleum was used to derive isopropyl alcohol from petroleum. Since then, petroleum has been the source of almost all the isopropyl alcohol used in industrialized nations. Other than in medicine, it has numerous uses, for instance, as an airplane wing and car windshield de-icer and as an industrial solvent. As a precursor of acetone, it served as the basis for the nascent synthetic fiber industry: Rayon is made from acetate, which became the principal product of acetone once the demand for explosives subsided. Petroleum thus replaced cellulose as the chief raw material for synthetic fibers. Acetate also is derived from acetylene, another petroleum derivative.

Ethylene: Uses and Hazards

In a similar vein, there are other whole families of chemicals derived from basic crude oil. Ethylene, one such raw material, has the greatest number of uses. It is obtained from ethane, which is abundant in crude petroleum and can be obtained by several other ways, including cracking. Ethylene reacts with oxygen to form ethylene oxide, which has a number of uses. It is used in practically every hospital in this country as a sterilizing gas for surgical instruments, endotracheal tubes, and other items too sensitive to be autoclaved. Ethylene oxide is a very reactive substance, and human exposure to it is hazardous. It is an irritant to the eyes, nose, throat, respiratory tract, and gastrointestinal tract, causing peculiar taste sensations. It causes central nervous system depression, as do many organic compounds. Heavy exposures result in pulmonary edema; degenerative changes in the lungs, liver, and kidneys; and death. Ethylene oxide combines with water to form the radiator antifreeze fluid, ethylene glycol.

Ethylene glycol (and other glycols) are heavy liquids with a sweet taste that are excellent solvents for water-insoluble substances, such as some drugs. Unfortunately, ethylene glycol is extremely toxic (Swinyard, 1975). In 1938, there was a mass poisoning of consumers of a new product: an elixir of sulfanilamide compound that consisted of 8 percent sulfanilamide (one of the best and most widely used antibiotics of the pre-penicillin era) in 72 percent diethylene glycol and 20 percent flavoring and water (Arena, 1979). One hundred and five patients who had consumed from one to four teaspoons of the new compound died. The public outrage that followed the incident resulted in the U.S. Food and Drug Administration (FDA) being given the task to assure that drugs marketed in the United States are safe (only many years later was the FDA given the mandate to ascertain that drugs are also effective).

Glycols are metabolized *in vivo* to oxalic acid, which is toxic to the central nervous system and the kidneys and causes anemia and metabolic acidosis. Treatment, interestingly, is ethyl alcohol, which blocks the metabolic pathway of the glycol by competition, thus forcing its excretion in its unmetabolized harmless state. Even though ethylene glycol poisoning is rare now, cases continue to occur, chiefly among children who mistake the sweet-tasting, brightly colored liquid for a soft drink, or among suicidal individuals. Another reported mechanism of ethylene glycol toxicity occurs in intubated patients in hospitals. Ethylene oxide residue on the endotracheal tube sterilized with that gas combines with water in the respiratory secretions to form ethylene glycol in the trachea. This has been reported as a cause of tracheal injury in the anesthesiology literature.

Ethylene has many other uses, far too many to discuss here; however, the structure of this molecule enabled it to help usher in the "Plastic Age" in which we live. When ethylene is bonded to itself, it forms a polymer, polyethylene, a plastic with many uses. Ethylene combined with a chlorine atom forms polyvinyl chloride monomer, a carcinogen that has become an occupational hazard and is discussed in Chapter 6. When polymerized, this monomer forms polyvinyl chloride (PVC), a very strong plastic that is familiar to nearly everyone. Indeed, these and other plastics have been called the leading products of the petrochemical industry for the past 50 years.

The Prevalence of Petrochemicals

The vast array of petrochemicals is stunning to anyone trying to learn about chemicals and their role in modern life and ecosystems. Thousands of new chemicals are synthesized yearly, not only in the petrochemical industry, but from coal, natural gas, and agricultural products (corn, soybeans, and cane sugar). Many of these compounds are synthetic, meaning they do not exist in nature. Thus, no living thing having been exposed to them, their impact on the environment is unpredictable, as are their effects on human health. Literally hundreds of new chemicals (of the thousands synthesized) are introduced into industry or commercial use each year. Most of these are beneficial in some way, although many uses are of controversial or marginal benefit. Occasionally, however, there is a product put into widespread use that is so harmful it can only be described as a disaster. Such products are the polychlorinated biphenyls and the polybrominated biphenyls, subjects of the next section. However, before reading on, consider an issue that environmentally minded health professionals may find worth pondering. Nearly every hospital now administers drugs and intravenous fluids to its patients via disposable plastic bags, tubes, and syringes. These replaced similar equipment made of glass, which is generally considered chemically inert. The change to disposable products decreased the risk of hospital-acquired infections for the patients but increased the risks of parenteral exposures to plastics and plasticizers (chemicals added to plastics to make them more pliant). In addition, there may be interactions with the drugs and electrolytes that are being administered via these plastic systems.

We must consider the possible effects of this. What are the potential long-term risks for children, obstetric patients and their babies, anephric patients, and others? One can go beyond the bounds of the hospital and ask what the health effects on the community are of disposing tons of plastic from hospitals, rather than using the recyclable equipment the plastic replaced. (The issue of chemical waste will be discussed later.) These questions are largely unanswered; indeed, they are largely unasked.

HALOGENATED HYDROCARBONS

Halogenated hydrocarbons are a rather large and varied group of compounds, nearly none of which exist in nature. As their name implies, they have in common their chemical composition: carbon, hydrogen, sometimes oxygen, and a halogen, usually chlorine or bromine (or both) and occasionally fluorine. They vary from simple to complex in structure. Their uses include solvents (trichloroethylene), pesticides (DDT), medicine (chloral hydrate), plastics (polyvinyl chloride), and others. Many of these compounds are toxic, and their use is strictly controlled (carbon tetrachloride, PCBs, and dibromochloropropane). We will focus on polychlorinated biphenyls (PCBs), not only because they are important compounds, but also because they serve as a kind of terrible model for many other compounds. However, one cannot separate a discussion of PCBs from one of dioxins or furans, which are unavoidable contaminants of PCBs and many other chlorinated aromatic hydrocarbons.

Dioxins

Dioxins have received considerable attention in the past few years (Whiteside, 1979) because they are also unavoidable contaminants of the chlorphenoxy herbicide, 2,4,5-trichlorophenoxyacetic acid (2,4,5-T). This compound usually was used in combination with 2,4-dichlorophenoxyacetic acid (2,4-D), which contains no dioxin. They were used to control growth of weeds along roads, utility rights of way, and commercial forests. However, their most controversial uses were as weapons in the Vietnam War. A combination of 2,4,5-T and 2,4-D, called Agent Orange, was sprayed by the U.S. Air Force in "Operation Ranch Hand" on jungles, trails, and rice paddies of Southeast Asia for years. The stated purposes of the spraying were to make it difficult for the Vietnamese to move men and material without detection through the thick overgrowth and to deny the rice crop to the Viet Cong and North Vietnamese Army. As a result of the spraying, thousands, if not millions, of American, Allied, Vietnamese, and other soldiers and Vietnamese civilian men, women, and children were exposed to Agent Orange and its dioxin. An estimated 11 million pounds of herbicide containing 220 pounds of dioxin were sprayed (Schneider, 1979). Because of the lack of scientific data and a number of confounding variables, measuring the effects, if any, on the Vietnamese population has been difficult. In this country, Vietnam-era veterans, thousands of whom were exposed, have petitioned the Veterans Administration to evaluate them for health effects due to their exposure. To date, the only health effect that has been linked firmly to dioxin is chloracne. The many other health effects noted (skin rashes, fatigue, decreased fertility, emotional disorders, cancers, liver disorders, nervous disorders, and others) require further epidemiologic studies, some of which are ongoing.

The first major study of American Vietnam-era veterans was published in 1984 by a team of epidemiologists from the Centers for Disease Control (Erickson, Mulinare, McClain, Fitch, James, McClearn, & Adams, 1984). Using a case-control study involving more than 10,000 families, they assessed the veterans' risks for fathering infants with major birth defects. The Metropolitan Atlanta Congenital Defects Program, a registry of congenital malformations, provided the data base from which the team identified cases; controls were selected from the more than 300,000 live-born infants in Atlanta from 1968 through 1980. The parents were located and interviewed; veteran status and exposure to Agent Orange were assessed both by subjective recall and by a search of military records. The analysis did not produce evidence that veterans had any greater risk of fathering children with serious structural defects than did other men. Results from other studies are forthcoming. An important public-health challenge will be to present these politically sensitive results in a fair, compassionate, and yet scientifically convincing way.

Dioxins are extremely toxic, extremely stable compounds about which there is much that is unknown. The dioxin that contaminates 2,4,5-T is 2,3,7,8-tetrachlorodibenzo-p dioxin (TCDD) (see Figure 3–1). It is one of the most toxic substances known. Toxicity is usually expressed as the amount that constitutes a lethal dose for 50 percent (LD_{50}) of a particular species of animal. The LD_{50} for TCDD is 0.6 micrograms per kilogram (μg/kg) for male guinea pigs. Compare this with the LD_{50} of 2,4,5-T of 381 milligrams per kilogram (mg/kg) for the same species and sex—a difference of more than 600,000 times! The Agent Orange used in Vietnam is thought to have been heavily contaminated with TCDD. The use of 2,4,5-T has been banned in this country, although 2,4-D, which does not contain TCDD, is still in use.

PCBs

PCBs, as mentioned earlier, are semisynthetic oils. They were made from biphenyl, a naturally occurring compound extracted from petroleum. The biphenyl is chlorinated at any or all of its car-

Figure 3-1   Chemical Structure of Tetrachlorodibenzodioxin (TCDD)

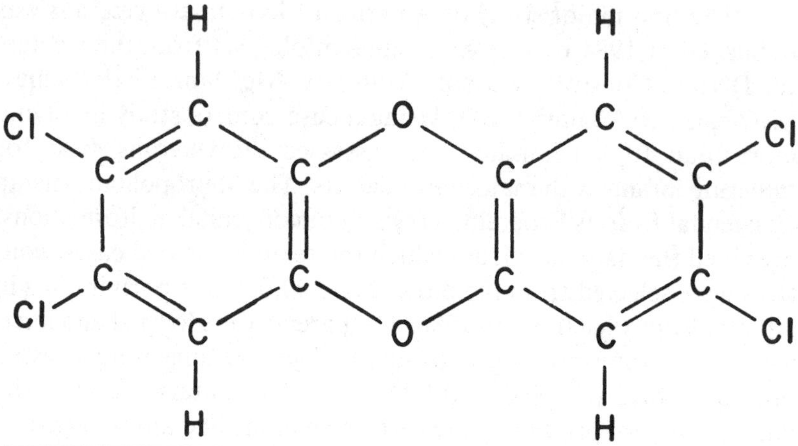

bon atoms (see Figure 3-2) in the presence of a catalyst (usually iron). The result is a mixture of PCBs that are heavy, nonflammable, stable oils with high boiling points and low electrical conductivity. These properties made them ideal coolants for electrical transformers, as well as superior hydraulic fluids, stone-cutting oils, and heat transfer fluids. They had a number of other uses such as plasticizers and dye carriers in carbonless multiple-copy office forms.

Figure 3-2   Chemical Structure of Polyhalogenated Biphenyls (PBBs and PCBs)

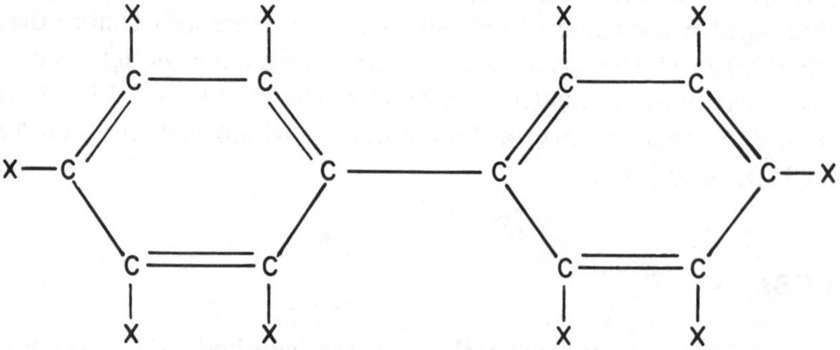

X = H AND Br OR Cl

Much of what we know about the toxicity of PCBs comes from an incident in Japan in 1968 (Higuchi, 1976). Rice oil is very popular there for cooking, and manufacture of this oil requires pressing rice bran at high pressures. This generates considerable heat. PCBs were used as the cooling fluid in this process. Clearly there was a leak or cross-connection in the system at one rice oil plant, for the oil became heavily contaminated with PCBs. Within a few weeks, over 1000 consumers of the oil were ill. The illness, which the local people called Yusho (or oil sickness), was characterized by chloracne (mild to severe acneiform eruption); hyperpigmentation of skin, nails, and conjunctival and mucous membranes; liver disease (including necrosis); fatigue; headache; menstrual disorders; palpebral edema and meibomian hypersecretion; birth defects (usually hyperpigmentation); and other findings. Breast-fed infants not exposed to the oil directly also suffered, indicating that mothers were passing the contamination on to their babies via their milk. Follow-up studies showed that the PCBs were contaminated with polychlorinated dibenzofurans (similar to dioxins). These probably played a significant role in the toxicity. Laboratory study indicates that PCBs cause hepatocellular carcinoma in rats. Epidemiologists and clinicians continue to monitor the Yusho victims to learn the long-term effects of the disease in humans. This incident caused the Japanese government to ban the production, import, or export of PCBs in 1972.

The more PCBs are studied, the more we understand that the Yusho incident is unique only in that the exposure was very high. Exposure to PCBs is virtually universal in industrialized countries. Almost all residents of the United States have detectable amounts of PCBs in their bodies. The chemical stability and fat solubility of PCBs causes them to bioaccumulate through the food chain.

A typical example of environmental contamination might start with a discarded power transformer from a farm or a factory. There are literally thousands of such transformers currently in use, each containing up to a few hundred gallons of PCBs. The discarded transformer sits outdoors until it corrodes and the PCB oil leaks out. Rain eventually washes the oil into a creek. Since PCBs are heavier than water, they stay at the bottom of the creek bed where they may be taken up by microorganisms, eaten by bottom-feeding fish, or washed along with the current.

This scenario has been documented over and over again. In a flagrant example, the General Electric Company, under permits granted by state and federal authorities, dumped 30 pounds of chlorinated hydrocarbons a day from a capacitor plant into the Hudson River in New York State, resulting in a build-up of approximately 600 tons of PCBs in the river basin by 1975. The problem was discovered by government inspectors who found high PCB levels in fish samples taken from commercial fishing boats. Bass and perch averaged 62 to 135 parts per million (ppm) of PCBs, which was well above the then-current U.S. Food and Drug Administration limit of five ppm. The limit since has been lowered to two ppm.

Consumers of fresh-water fish in North America are at high risk of absorbing PCBs into their bodies, where they are stored in the fat. The biological half-life of PCBs is years, and no one knows what the long-term risks of PCB bioaccumulation are. The problem is also very serious in the Great Lakes and Upper Chesapeake Bay regions, where PCBs have polluted the fish and crabs to levels well above the FDA limits. Some health authorities have recommended against eating any fresh-water fish for this reason (ocean fish do not seem to be similarly contaminated).

Significant controversies exist in these regions for lactating mothers. Some surveys in Michigan reveal PCB concentrations in human breast milk that exceed the FDA tolerance limit of 1.5 ppm for cow's milk. Thus far, the best advice for such mothers is to continue breast feeding, because breast milk is known to be the best milk for babies (with a possible exception being mothers with unique or unduly high PCB exposures, such as those in occupational settings). However, organizations such as the State Health Department, the La Leche League, and the American Academy of Pediatrics are keeping a careful watch on this and related issues. It behooves health professionals to keep current on these issues in order to counsel patients and parents (Rogan, 1980). Prevention is essential here, because there is no known treatment for PCB poisoning or any way to enhance PCB excretion. Elimination of further exposure, whether it be on the job or in the diet, is of paramount importance.

An illustration of how ubiquitous and insidious PCB contamination is involves an incident in 1979. An unused transformer at a hog slaughterhouse in Montana was punctured accidentally. The PCBs leaked out and entered the plant's recycling system for grease, waste meats, and the like. The waste was sold to a large chicken farm in Idaho in the form of meatmeal protein supplement for chicken feed. Over the next several months the chickens laid eggs laced with PCBs. The eggs were sold to groceries all over the western United States and to commercial food processers such as bakeries and mayonnaise makers. The contamination was discovered, and literally millions of dollars worth of food had to be recalled from across the United States to be destroyed. Human absorption of PCBs was documented by correlating egg consumption with breast milk PCB levels in the small town where the chicken farm was located (Drotman, Baxter, Liddle, et al., 1983). The incident pointed out the need for continued vigilance and chemical surveillance of the food supply. There is no doubt that similar incidents go undetected.

PESTICIDES: ECONOMIC POISONS

The discussion of chlorinated hydrocarbons leads easily to one of pesticides because one of the most important groups of pesticides has been the chlorinated hydrocarbons, or, as they are usually termed, organochlorine insecticides. This group includes DDT (see Figure 3–3).

Defining "pesticide" can be controversial. It depends on what one considers a "pest." Generally, pests include insects, worms, rodents, weeds, and fungi; but even this list can stir debate. Which plants are weeds? Which insects are beneficial? Virtually all households in the United States use pesticides of one kind or another. Uses

Figure 3–3   Chemical Structure of Dichlorodiphenyl Trichloroethane (DDT)

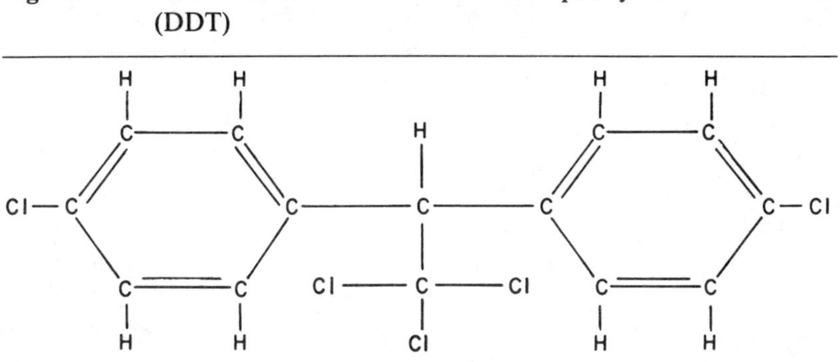

include termite treatment of the ground around foundations, moth-balls, bug sprays, cockroach and rat poisons, and flea and tick pro-tectors for pets.

Finding suitable agents to use as pesticides is analogous to the search for the first antibiotics: seeking the "magic bullet," as Paul Ehrlich termed it, as he pursued the first chemotherapeutic agent for treating syphilis in 1910. The "magic bullets" of pesticides must be lethal to the pest, safe for nontarget organisms, and inexpensive. There is, of course, no pesticide that completely meets all the re-quirements. Pests have developed resistance to many agents; all pesticides are toxic to nontarget organisms to some degree; and all cost money to manufacture, apply, and dispose of when they are no longer wanted. These are problems society has been unwilling to confront until very recently.

As mentioned earlier in this chapter, DDT was viewed as a great step forward in 1939 when its insecticidal properties were dis-covered. Because of World War II, its immediate uses were as a delousing powder for refugees and soldiers and, in an oil suspen-sion, for controlling malaria-carrying mosquitoes in war areas. How-ever, the chief market for DDT was to be agricultural. Perhaps the largest users of DDT were cotton growers (to control the boll weevil).

Cotton continues to be the source of demand for much of the production of all types of pesticides. The U.S. Department of Agri-culture estimated national production of pesticides to be about 100 million pounds in 1945. By 1975, the production rose exponen-tially to 1.6 billion pounds, nearly 8 pounds for every person in the country. (To be sure, much of the American production of pesti-cides and other chemicals is exported; however, the responsible use of many of these agents in underdeveloped countries is open to question.)

Pesticides replaced traditional pest control strategies such as crop rotation, tilling agricultural wastes to deprive pests of out-of-season sustenance, and use of the pests' natural enemies. However, widespread resistance among the pests has caused new research into the usefulness of combining the old strategies with chemical pesti-cides. This now is termed "integrated pest management" and is viewed with hope by the environmental and agricultural communi-ties.

Organochlorine Pesticides

This class of pesticides includes familiar names such as DDT, chlordane, toxaphene, and lindane, among many others. However, almost none of them are generally available for use. An exception is lindane, which, in addition to its use in the fields, is prescribed commonly under the brand name Kwell® for human lice and scabies infestations.

The organochlorines are neurotoxins. In high doses, they disrupt axonic transmission of nerve impulses in both the central and peripheral nervous systems. Human exposure to this class of agents may produce excitability, headache, disorientation, paresthesias, convulsions, coma, and death (Morgan, 1977). If ingested, severe nausea and vomiting commonly result. Some of the organochlorines are hepatotoxins, especially endrin, which is probably the most toxic member of this class of pesticides. The prognosis for patients poisoned with this class of agents is generally good. Fatal cases are usually the result of massive doses (such as in suicides or accidental ingestions among children). Treatment principles include (1) preventing further absorption by inducing vomiting (with ipecac), gastric lavage, and oral administration of activated charcoal; (2) supporting respiration by administering oxygen, clearing the airway of secretions, and assisting pulmonary ventilation, if necessary; and (3) controlling convulsions with diazepam or pentobarbital. These principles of treatment apply to many acutely poisoned patients, not just those who have ingested organochlorines.

The use of organochlorines has declined considerably in the past decade because of severe regulatory restrictions placed on their use in this and some other countries. The restrictions were put into effect for several reasons. The organochlorines are highly persistent in the environment, just as the PCBs are. Chlordane placed in the earth around residences to protect them against subterranean termites has been found in virtually the same concentrations 10 years after application. Many of the organochlorines were not placed in the ground, but on crops; thus they ran off the fields in the rain. In streams and ponds they are taken up by microorganisms, which in turn are consumed by other organisms. Thus, they enter the food chain in two ways: as residues on animal feed or human food crops and in organisms that are taken up by other organisms.

Although DDT was banned at the end of 1972, except for export (usually for use in malaria control) and some public health and medical uses (such as controlling bats to prevent rabies), it continues to be found in the environment. The most flagrant example of this is in Triana, Alabama, where residents have the highest concentrations of DDT in their bodies (serum and fat) ever recorded (Kreiss, Zack, Kimbrough, et al., 1981). Triana has the misfortune to be downstream from the Redstone Arsenal, which had a DDT plant on its premises. Over the life of the plant, which closed in the 1970s, great quantities of DDT were dumped into the Triana River (reasons for dumping might include slight misformulations and others). The DDT became concentrated in fish living in the river, which were, in turn, an important component of the diet of the poor black people of Triana. They are now the subjects of study because of their unusual body burdens.

The persistence of DDT in the environment; its bioaccumulation, which has resulted in the near-extinction of a number of bird species (notably, several kinds of eagles and the brown pelican); and the discovery that it produces cancer in laboratory rats and mice culminated in the near-total ban. Unfortunately, there continues to be a black market for DDT because some farmers continue to find it useful. As social scientists know, it is difficult to enforce a ban on nearly anything in a free society. Even without illicit use, DDT and the other organochlorines will continue to be in the food chain for the foreseeable future, and virtually all people in the United States will continue to concentrate it in their fatty tissues, even before birth, because all of these chemicals cross the placenta (Curley, Copeland, & Kimbrough, 1969).

Organophosphorus Pesticides

Organophosphorus pesticides are probably the most widely and extensively used group of insecticides. Agents of this class include parathion, malathion, chlorpyrifos, diazinon, and many others. They all have a similar chemical structure (phosphate esters) and a nearly identical mode of action. They phosphorylate, i.e., nearly irreversibly inhibit, the enzyme cholinesterase. Cholinesterase normally detoxifies acetylcholine. The build-up of acetylcholine that results from exposure to an organophosphate causes continual stimulation of the central, somatic, and parasympathetic nervous systems. These agents are absorbed readily through the skin and the respiratory and gastrointestinal tracts. They produce a predictable variety of effects: parasympathetic effects include constriction of the pupils, sweating and salivation, vomiting and diarrhea, cough and increased respiratory secretions, and possibly pulmonary edema. Somatic effects include lack of coordination, muscle twitching and weakness, and paralysis. Central nervous system effects include confused mental state, ataxia, convulsions, coma, respiratory depression, and death (Morgan, 1977). The research that produced the model for this class of compounds was carried out in Germany during World War II. The goal of the research was to develop chemical warfare agents — commonly known as "nerve gas."

Except for malathion and a few others, these agents are rather toxic to mammals as well as insects. The reason for malathion's exception is its rapid metabolism by the mammalian liver. However, high doses can overcome this protection and cause all the effects listed previously. Reasons for the persistent popularity of organophosphates are their great variety, which can be used by farmers to reduce the emergence of resistant strains of insects, and their biodegradability. All agents of this class are broken down in the environment or in animals or humans exposed to them. Subclinical exposure to organophosphates can be measured in humans by determining the level of cholinesterase activity in the plasma, or more accurately, in the red blood cells. Decreases in cholinesterase activity indicate exposure has occurred.

Treatment for mild exposures is simply to stop the exposure. For example, agricultural workers or florists might be taken off the job for a short while until the agent is metabolized and their cholinesterase activity rebounds. Naturally, preventive measures should be adopted, such as wearing impervious gloves or other protective clothing to decrease skin absorption. Respiratory exposure can be minimized by avoiding areas where spraying is going on.

More severe exposures can be treated specifically with atropine and pralidoxime. Atropine does not restore the cholinesterase but does protect against the excessive acetylcholine concentrations until cholinesterase activity returns. Thus, the principle of treatment is to stabilize the patient with atropine and supportive measures (see previous section) until the toxin is metabolized. This may take up to 10 days in very severe poisonings, but the prognosis with adequate treatment is quite favorable. Pralidoxime does regenerate inhibited cholinesterase and is a useful adjunct to therapy.

Carbamate Pesticides

In general, carbamates are less toxic than organophosphates, although symptoms of acute poisoning are essentially identical. Members of this class include aldicarb (Temik®), a systemic agent taken up by the plant and stored in the foliage or fruit; propoxur (Baygon®); and carbaryl (Sevin®). These are also very popular among farmers, gardeners, and foresters.

Because the carbamate inactivation of cholinesterase is reversible, laboratory determinations of cholinesterase activity can err on the side of being normal. Another method of testing for carbamate exposure is to measure betanaphthal in the urine. The presence of this metabolic product of the carbamates in more than trace amounts generally indicates carbamate intoxication. Clinical carbamate poisoning is nearly identical to that seen with organophosphates except that carbamates do not penetrate the central nervous system very well and thus produce only limited effects there. Treatment is identical to that of the organophosphates except that pralidoxime is not used because reversal of cholinesterase inhibition may occur too rapidly and be harmful.

Other Pesticides

There are literally thousands of other pesticides in addition to the ones discussed already. They range from paraquat, an herbicide that has gained notoriety from governmental efforts to use it on marijuana fields; to pentachlorophenol, a wood preservative used in log homes; to warfarin; a commonly prescribed blood anticoagulant used as a rodenticide; to arsenic compounds used as insecticides and herbicides (Morgan, 1977).

When pesticides are manufactured, used, and disposed of in a responsible and thoughtful manner, they are usually safe. However, this is not always the case. Some are brought to market before their toxicity is known. Workers may be exposed to the toxins during their manufacture and be at risk for health effects about which they have no knowledge. This is precisely what happened to employees of Oxy Chemicals, who worked in production of dibromochloropropane (DBCP), a very popular and persistent nematocide (worm killer) (Whorton, Krauss, Marshall, & Milby, 1977). A group of male workers, by talking with one another, discovered they had become infertile. Later research confirmed that DBCP caused their inability to father children. The use of DBCP is now regulated, but much of it persists in soil and is percolating down to water tables from Hawaii to Florida. Many wells in farming areas are now contaminated with DBCP. The long-term effects on humans of DBCP in minute exposures are unknown.

Smokers of marijuana may be exposed unknowingly to paraquat. It is extremely irritating, and symptoms of inhalation may include sore throat, nosebleed, and cough. Severe exposure may result in pneumonitis, pulmonary edema, and death; but paraquat is so irritating that it is unlikely anyone would or could inhale that much. Severe poisonings usually have occurred as a result of ingestion. Fortunately, this herbicide is not generally available. No cases of paraquat-associated lung disease have been documented among American smokers of marijuana.

Pentachlorophenol (PCP) has been used as a wood preservative on utility poles and railroad ties for decades. The recent popularity of prefabricated log homes has caused some concern since the logs are preserved by dipping them in PCP, a persistent chlorinated hydrocarbon. PCP is a metabolic uncoupler; large exposures could produce malignant hyperthermia, especially in an already hot environment. However, the effects of long term (life-long for children raised in log homes) exposure to relatively low levels of PCP are unknown. Recent investigation has documented that absorption of PCP does occur among residents of such homes.

The litany goes on and on. Despite abuses of the past and present, there is hope for the future. Rachel Carson deserves considerable credit for bringing the pesticide situation to our national attention in her now classic work, *Silent Spring* (1962). Since the publication of this book, the federal Environmental Protection Agency (EPA) has been established (in 1970), and most states also regulate the use of pesticides.

In general, the EPA licenses pesticides for use on certain crops (see Chapter 8). The Food and Drug Administration (FDA) sets tolerance levels for concentrations of residues of pesticides (and other substances, such as PCBs) in food and food packaging. The U.S. Department of Agriculture (USDA) encourages integrated pest management and sponsors research on pest management control programs.

The formulation of environmentally sound and sensibly enforced regulations remains a challenge for the American political and public health systems. It runs counter to American tradition and the free enterprise system not to allow farmers to use the cheapest and best agent they can, in whatever concentration they choose, to bring their most bountiful harvest to market each year. Educating farmers, and indeed individual households, that pesticides are biologically active agents with potentially wide-ranging effects is where the challenge lies. The development of a resistant strain of insects on one farm this year may mean resistance on all farms next year, with loss of crops for all. This lesson has been learned the hard way in many areas. Irresponsibly spraying or dumping excess pesticide where it may run off into a reservoir or river used as a drinking water source or percolate down to the water table adds to the body burden of all those exposed and in severe cases may cause an epidemic of poisoning in nontarget wild animals as well as people and/or livestock. As the population grows and water and food supply systems become more complex and more interdependent, the potential for disastrous exposures increases, unless safeguards are put in place beforehand.

INORGANIC COMPOUNDS

Until now, nearly all the substances discussed have been organic compounds or synthetic derivatives of them. However, many highly toxic agents exist among the inorganics: Lead, mercury, and arsenic have proven to be significant pollutants and toxins. Asbestos is also an inorganic substance, a mineral fiber, that has very toxic properties probably due to its physical, rather than chemical, activity in the body.

Many other metals are potentially toxic; however, some, such as calcium, sodium, potassium, and magnesium, are better discussed in physiology texts because they play key roles in human metabolic processes. Aluminum, zinc, and tin are common components of food storage and cooking containers and usually are considered nontoxic. More attention is being paid to aluminum, however, because high levels have been found in patients with certain mental disorders such as Alzheimer's disease (premature senility). The clinical significance of this finding is currently unknown. Copper is usually toxic only to those with special susceptibility known as Wilson's disease, a genetic disorder of copper metabolism. Iron is an essential nutrient, but is toxic in large doses.

There are some toxicities that many metals have in common. One of these is termed metal fume fever (Dreisbach, 1977). Exposure to freshly generated oxides of zinc or many other metals results in polymyalgia (generalized muscle pains), fever, chills, headache, nausea and vomiting, and weakness. The treatment consists of stopping exposure to the fumes, rest, and aspirin. The pathophysiology of the disease is unknown, but chronic poisoning does not seem to occur. This condition is rather common simply because so many people are exposed to welding fumes on their jobs or in hobby work.

Because there are so many elements and compounds, each with its own routes of exposure, metabolism, toxicology, and epidemiology, only two of the more important metals will be covered in this chapter: lead and mercury. Technically, it is incorrect to consider these elements strictly as inorganic chemicals because they are incorporated into organic compounds as well and both become more toxic to humans than in their inorganic state.

Lead

Some of the past history of lead was discussed at the beginning of the chapter. Its more recent history is equally fascinating. Because it is common, used in so many ways in the home and the workplace, and so toxic, lead has been the subject of intense study (Needleman, 1980). Even so, there is much we do not know about its relation to human health.

Lead is extremely toxic. Clinical toxicity can occur in adults who absorb as little as 0.5 milligrams per day (much less for organic lead). Children are more sensitive to the toxic effects of lead than are adults. Many children have suffered and, tragically, continue to suffer lead toxicity from ingestion of lead-based paint. It is completely preventable and has received considerable attention, but it continues to occur in this country.

Lead-based paint was used inside many homes until Congress passed the Lead-Based Paint Poisoning Prevention Act in 1971. Since then, lead has not been added to paint used inside residences or on furniture or toys. Such paint still is used industrially, outside buildings, and on automobiles. However, such laws only truly protect new housing units. Millions of older dwellings still have many layers of lead-based paint. When small children see the colorful flakes of paint on windowsills or around baseboards, they are attracted to them and many put the flakes in their mouths and swallow them.

Although paint ingestion is the primary source of lead exposure for children (due to the high concentration of lead found in such paint), it is far from being the only source of exposure. Lead is encountered in air, water, and soil. It is used as a gasoline additive (tetraethyl lead) to improve the fuel's burning characteristics (decreases engine "knock"). Thus, lead is one component of air pollution, particularly in cities. It soon settles in urban soils and is taken up by vegetation, including food crops in gardens. Lead is found in many workplaces, especially mines, soldering shops, radiator and battery shops, and a host of others. A worker can bring lead dust home on workclothes and spread the toxin throughout the household, to spouse and children. Nearly everyone, especially those living in cities, has absorbed some lead into their bodies. Although there is no conclusive evidence that the levels usually detected are harmful, there is support for the theory that subclinical exposure to lead does influence childhood behavior disorders (such as hyperactivity) and intelligence. There is no evidence that a small amount of lead is beneficial, as there is for a number of other trace metals.

Lead is absorbed via the gastrointestinal and respiratory tracts. It also can be absorbed through the skin, but this route is less important. It enters the circulation and is deposited in bones, brain and peripheral nervous tissue, and bone marrow. X-rays of long bones may show "lead lines" at the metaphysis. Lead poisoning can mimic virtually any encephalopathy—an ominous sign. It may present as a peripheral neuropathy—classically, a "wrist drop" or flaccid paralysis of the wrist. However, the diagnosis is made most frequently because of lead's effect on red blood cell formation. Lead interferes with several enzymes necessary for hemoglobin synthesis. This results in anemia, decreased reticulocyte count, and basophilic stippling of the red cells. A commonly used screening test for lead poisoning in children is also a test for anemia (erythrocyte protoporphyrin, or EP). An EP level of over 50 micrograms per deciliter (μg/dl) indicates either iron deficiency anemia or lead toxicity (CDC, 1978). The two conditions then must be distinguished. This can be done by measuring blood lead.

The current standard or "upper limit of normal" for blood lead in children is 30 μg/dl (CDC, 1978); for adults the occupational standard is 60 μg/dl. For individuals whose blood levels exceed the standards, further exposure must be avoided. Unfortunately, this is not always done; children and their parents may be ignorant of the threat to their health, and workers may fear employer reprisals if they complain about undue lead exposure. However, the lead problem has decreased considerably, due to increased recognition and to screening programs for children and houses in most larger cities. There also have been recent decreases in blood lead levels attributed to reduced use of lead as a gasoline additive (CDC, 1982). Although this cannot yet be considered a public health triumph, at least the problem is not getting significantly worse, as it had been for most of this century.

Fortunately, there is treatment for lead poisoning; however, the pathology, especially nervous system disorders, is not reversible in all cases. Children with encephalopathy nearly always suffer sequelae. Chelating agents such as EDTA (ethylene diamine tetraacetic acid), BAL (British anti-Lewisite), and penicillamine mobilize lead from its storage sites in the body and cause its excretion via the kidneys. This therapy requires close medical monitoring, usuallly in a hospital. The duration of therapy depends on the amount of lead absorbed. One of the most important principles in rehabilitating lead-poisoned patients, especially children, is never to send the patient back into a lead-contaminated environment. This is one condition where prevention is paramount.

Mercury

Mercury is far less common than lead, but it has been involved in a number of important incidents, such as the Minimata Bay tragedy referred to at the beginning of this chapter (Smith & Smith, 1975). It is a significant water pollutant in several places. Mercury is used in medicine and dentistry in a variety of ways, so members of those professions should be aware of its toxicity.

Mercury is found in three chemical forms (in increasing order of toxicity): elemental mercury (the only metal that is liquid at room temperature), inorganic salts, and organic compounds (alkyl compounds are more toxic than phenyl compounds). Metallic mercury — the type found in thermometers, sphygmomanometers, and other instruments — is not absorbed from the gastrointestinal tract and therefore not very hazardous if swallowed (thus, the major danger from a broken oral or rectal thermometer is the broken glass). However, it is absorbed from the lungs, and mercury vapor is hazardous, especially if it is heated. Thus, thermometers broken inside infant incubators can present severe problems for the babies inside when the spilled mercury leaks down to the heating units (McLaughlin, Telzrow, & Scott, 1980). Metallic mercury is mixed vigorously with silver to form the amalgam dentists use to fill teeth. If the amalgamator is open, significant mercury exposure may result. Mercury also is released when the dentist carves and shapes the amalgam. This presents more of an occupational hazard to the dentist and dental assistants, whose exposures are prolonged, than to the patient, whose exposure is intermittent.

Inorganic mercury salts such as mercuric choloride once were used in medicine as antiseptics. These have been replaced by equally effective, less toxic agents. Inorganics are industrial pollutants. They can be transformed by bacteria to the more toxic organic mercurials and enter the food chain. Fresh-water fish are particularly at risk for such contamination, especially those near chlor-alkali plants and paper plants where mercuric chloride is used as a bleach for the paper and is subsequently discharged into the water.

Organic mercury compounds continue to be used as fungicides on seeds for crops. From time to time, people have consumed the seeds rather than plant them. In one severe outbreak in New Mexico (Pierce, 1972), a family consumed a pig that had eaten the seeds,

and other outbreaks of acute mercury poisoning have resulted.
Mercury is a nervous system toxin, causing tremors, ataxia, irritability, slurred speech, dementia, blindness, and death. Mercury was used in processing felt for hats in the last century; persons employed in this trade were so often intoxicated by the mercury that they became known as "mad hatters." Although treatment in the form of chelation therapy may be offered, it is not usually effective. This is yet another disease where prevention is the only viable approach.

THE PERSONAL ENVIRONMENT

One goal of this chapter is to make readers more aware of their personal environment. Readers, it is hoped, will examine their own living, learning, and working environments, including what substances are present and what exposures are possible. They then will determine what hazards, if any, may exist and what can be done to prevent them.

A multitude of questions can be raised about the basic personal environment. For example, with our effort to conserve energy, we have sealed and insulated our homes and offices (see Chapter 5). Pollutants such as carbon monoxide; carbon dioxide; and oxides of nitrogen from cigarettes, woodburning stoves, kerosene heaters, and fireplaces may render the indoor environment hazardous. Chemicals such as methanol from spirit duplicators and multicarbon compounds from photoduplicators may pollute offices. Insulation can be hazardous. We have known for years that asbestos fibers cause asbestosis (an obstructive lung disease) and mesothelioma (a particularly virulent form of cancer), but it is still present in many homes, schools, and workplaces (International Agency for Research on Cancer [IARC], 1977). Urea formaldehyde foam has been used as an insulator for mobile homes and (usually) older stationary homes. It can release formaldehyde gas, a mucous membrane irritant and allergen that has been shown recently to produce cancer in rats and mice. Medical workers exposed to this chemical in laboratories are all too frequently unaware of its potential hazards. The federal Consumer Product Safety Commission has banned urea formaldehyde foam, and the National Institute for Occupational Health and Safety has set recommended limits on occupational exposures to formalde-hyde. Both these actions, however, are in dispute, and their final impacts are unclear for now.

The quality of drinking water may be imperiled by natural deposits of nitrates or arsenic that may leach into wells. Irresponsibly used or disposed pesticides may drift into an aquifer; or a toxic waste dump may contaminate a watershed, reservoir, or river (National Research Council, 1977).

Many foods are altered by artificial ingredients and preserva-tives, as well as by their containers. Many cans, for instance, have seams soldered with lead. While the levels of lead found in the food are not thought to be dangerous, they are much lower in food in cans without lead. In many parts of the world (the tropics and to some extent the southern United States), natural contamination of some grains and legumes with fungi is a significant problem of food storage. One particular fungus, *Aspergillus flavus*, produces aflatox-in, one of the most potent liver carcinogens known. Some meats are preserved with nitrites and nitrates; bacon has been one ex-ample. When it is cooked, the nitrite combines with amino acids in the meat to form nitrosamines, which are potent carcinogens (IARC, 1978).

The significance of these conditions remains controversial, as do the actions that individuals, health professionals, and society should take in response to them.

THE COMMUNITY ENVIRONMENT

There is little a single individual can do about some of the issues just posed: Avoiding all risks, even if they are avoidable, is a poor solution; for most, such a life would not be worth living. Learning what the risks are, which ones are trivial and which ones demand action, is a productive activity. The tool that environmental health professionals use in identifying risk factors is epidemiology.

The basic principles of epidemiology were outlined in Chapter 1. Epidemiology as it is used to assess environmental hazards is some-what different from traditional infectious disease epidemiology. In the latter, many of the important variables are known: the incuba-tion period, the usual attack rate and case-fatality rate, the usual course of the illness, and other such parameters. In environmental studies, these variables are rarely known; in many cases, the diseases or syndromes are not even known. The latent (or incubation) period may be decades, as it is for some cancers. Exposure to the causative agent may not even be remembered by the patient. A single agent may cause multiple effects and have multiple interactions. For example, asbestos causes both asbestosis and mesothelioma of the lung pleura and abdominal pleura. The latency period may be 20 years or more (IARC, 1977).

In assessing exposures to multiple agents, as was done at Love Canal, New York, the task may be hopelessly complex (see Chapter 7). Long-term studies of the affected population continue. The only health effects thus far firmly associated with living near the dump are decreased birth weight and an increase in nonspecific birth defects.

There are many challenges in environmental and occupational health, and many still to be discovered. More become apparent almost daily, but, despite the many obstacles, careful studies are being done, awareness increases, and strategies for prevention are being devised and disseminated.

SOURCES OF INFORMATION

One of the difficulties in studying environmental health problems is obtaining accurate, reliable, current information. Although the popular press has played an important role in bringing environmental issues to the attention of the public, many stories have been needlessly alarming or, on the other hand, excessively toned down.

The standard medical literature is useful. Many public health and epidemiologic journals have taken an active interest in environmental health, such as the *American Journal of Public Health*, the *Journal of Pediatrics*, and the *Journal of the American Medical Association*. Standard toxicology texts and journals are useful.

Many federal agencies publish information on specific chemicals: The National Institute of Environmental Health Sciences publishes an excellent journal, *Environmental Health Perspectives*. The Environmental Protection Agency has sponsored a large amount of research in environmental health and protection. It has regional offices in 10 major cities across the country and issues numerous publications. The Centers for Disease Control publishes *Morbidity and Mortality Weekly Report.*

Many state and local health departments now have environmental health units, and many of these are sources of information for local problems.

Private agencies and industry associations publish magazines, newsletters, and information. Some of these are the Sierra Club, Environmental Defense Fund, Cousteau Society, Audubon Society, and Chemical Manufacturers Association. These sources may provide leads for further investigation.

For rapid consultations in an emergency, poison-control centers usually have information on chemicals, drugs, pesticides, metals, oils and solvents, household substances like soap and shoe polish, and many other chemicals and biological agents.

REFERENCES

Arena JM. 1979. *Poisoning*, 4th ed. Springfield, Ill.: Charles C Thomas. 218–219.

Carson R. 1962. *Silent Spring*. Boston: Houghton Mifflin.

Centers for Disease Control. 1978. *Preventing Lead Poisoning in Young Children*. Atlanta: USDHEW Publication No. 1978.

Centers for Disease Control. 1982. Blood-Lead Levels in U.S. Population. *Morbidity and Mortality Weekly Report* 31:132–133.

Curley A, Copeland F, Kimbrough RD. 1969. Chlorinated Hydrocarbon Insecticides in Organs of Stillborn and Blood of Newborn Babies. *Archives of Environmental Health* 19:628–632.

Davies E, Edmundson F, ed. 1972. *Epidemiology of DDT*. Mount Kisco, N.Y.: Futura Publishing.

Dreisbach H. 1977. *Handbook of Poisoning: Diagnosis and Treatment*, 9th ed. Los Altos, Calif.: Lange Medical Publications.

Drotman DP, Baxter PJ, Liddle JA, Brokopp CD, Skinner MD. 1983. Contamination of the Food Chain by Polychlorinated Biphenyls from a Broken Transformer. *Am J Pub Health* 73:290–292.

Erickson JD, Mulinare J, McClain PW, Fitch TG, James LM, McClearn AB, Adams MJ. 1984. Vietnam Veterans' Risks for Fathering Babies with Birth Defects. *JAMA* 252:903–912.

Ericson JE, Shirahata MS, Patterson CC. 1979. Skeletal Concentrations of Lead in Ancient Peruvians. *New England Journal of Medicine* 300:946–951.

Higuchi K, ed. 1976. *PCB Poisoning and Pollution*. New York: Academic Press.

International Agency for Research on Cancer. 1977. *IARC Monographs on the*

Evaluation of Carcinogenic Risk of Chemicals to Man: Asbestos. Vol. 14. Lyon: IARC.

International Agency for Research on Cancer. 1978. *IARC Monographs on the Evaluation of the Carcinogenic Risk of Chemicals to Humans: Some N-Nitroso Compounds.* Vol. 17. Lyon: IARC.

Kipling MD, Waldron HA. 1976. Polycyclic Aromatic Hydrocarbons in Mineral Oil, Tar, and Pitch, Excluding Petroleum Pitch. *Preventive Medicine* 5: 262–278.

Kreiss K, Zack MM, Kimbrough RD, Needham LL, Smrek AL, Jones BT. 1981. Cross-Sectional Study of a Community with exceptional Exposure to DDT. *JAMA* 245:1926–1930.

Mack RB. 1973. Lead in History. *Clinical Toxicology Bulletin* 3:37–44.

McLaughlin JF, Telzrow RW, Scott CM. 1980. Neonatal Mercury Vapor Exposure in an Infant Incubator. *Pediatrics* 66:988–990.

Meadows H, Meadows D, Randers J, Behrens W III. 1974. *The Limits to Growth: A Report for the Club of Rome's Project on the Predicament of Mankind*, 2nd ed. New York: Universe Books.

Morgan DP. 1977. *Recognition and Management of Pesticide Poisonings*, 2nd ed. Washington, D.C.: U.S. Government Printing Office.

National Research Council, Safe Drinking Water Committee. 1977. *Drinking Water and Health.* Washington, D.C.: National Academy of Sciences.

Needleman, HL, ed. 1980. *Low Level Lead Exposure: The Clinical Implications of Current Research.* New York: Raven Press.

Needleman HL, Gunnoe CE, Leviton A, et al. 1979. Deficits in Psychologic and Classroom Performance of Children with Elevated Lead Levels. *New England Journal of Medicine* 300:689–695.

Read M. 1966. *Culture, Health, and Disease: Social and Cultural Influences on Health Programmes in Developing Countries.* London: Tavistock Publications.

Rogan WJ. 1980. The Sources and Routes of Childhood Chemical Exposures. *The Journal of Pediatrics* 97:861–865.

Schneider MJ. 1979. *Persistent Poisons: Chemical Pollutants in the Environment.* New York: The New York Academy of Sciences.

Smith WE, Smith AM. 1975. *Minamata.* New York: Holt, Rinehart and Winston.

Waldron HA. 1973. Lead Poisoning in the Ancient World. *Medical History* 17: 391–399.

Whiteside, T. 1979. *The Pendulum and the Toxic Cloud: The Course of Dioxin Contamination.* New Haven: Yale University Press.

Whorton D, Krauss RM, Marshall S, Milby TH. 1977. Infertility in Male Pesticide Workers. *Lancet* 2:1259–1261.

Chapter 4

The Health Effects of Low-Level Ionizing Radiation

Herman T. Blumenthal

> It does not matter to human tissue whether it is irradiated in peace or in war, by atomic fallout, by radiation from industrial plants or transportation units, by x-ray machines, or by radium treatment. It is injured in precisely the same way by excessive radiation from whatever source. [Schubert & Lapp, 1958, p. 8]

Living matter has always been exposed to some degree of radioactivity from what is now called natural background radiation. Van Cleave (1968) points out that the soil, the rocks, the bricks and stones of dwellings, and the air we breathe all contribute to the radiation to which we are continually subjected. Internally, natural constituents of cells and tissues, such as carbon and potassium, may be radioactive; and radiations from extraterrestrial sources (cosmic rays) are inescapably on the earth's surface.

In retrospect, damage from ionizing radiation was first observed among the pitchblende miners in Saxony and Bohemia about 500 years ago, although these miners were believed to have died of so-called mountain illness after five to ten years of underground mining (Harting & Hesse, 1879). It was not until after Becquerel's discovery in 1896 that ionizing radiations are emitted from natural uranium that these deaths among pitchblende miners were recognized to be due to cancer of the lung caused by the inhalation of radioactive dusts from the ores associated with the pitchblende.

In less than a century, radioactivity created by human ingenuity has been added to natural background radiation. Much of the early information about the effects of radiation on living matter resulted from the personal experiences of some of the pioneers who first carried out experiments with radioactive materials. Schubert and Lapp (1958) recount events noted above, as well as others dating back to the turn of this century, which reveal that doctors, patients, and scientists have been injured by excessive exposure to radiation, particularly since 1896, following Roentgen's discovery of x-rays and the isolation of radium by the Curies. Only 23 days after Roentgen's discovery, Grubbe sought medical aid for serious radiation burns of the hands. Madame Curie later died of the delayed effects of radium damage, and her daughter Irene, who continued her mother's scientific pursuits, succumbed to radiation-induced leukemia. In March 1896, Thomas Alva Edison also was experimenting with x-ray tubes. When he experienced smarting of the eyes and one of his assistants suffered severe x-ray burns, he abandoned these studies.

There also were other early occupational exposures to radioactivity, with harmful effects. Perhaps the most notorious was the uncovering, after World War I, of the dangers of applying radioactive paint to the dials and faces of watches and other instruments to render them visible in the dark. Those who painted the dials, the luminizers, mostly young women, suffered severe and often fatal anemia and bone cancer as the result of the deposition of radioactive materials in their bones and marrow. By 1922, there were already estimates that 100 radiologists had died as a result of overexposure to x-rays.

The lessons of history continue to accumulate. One recent retrospective study (Peters, Mackay, & Buckley, 1980) compared peptic ulcer patients, who were treated between 1948 and 1960 with x-irradiation to the stomach to reduce gastric acidity, with an age- and sex-matched group treated by gastrectomy alone. Mortality rates began to diverge 10 years after treatment, with mortalities higher in the irradiated group. While this group showed an excess of deaths from cancer of the stomach, it showed, as well, an increase in deaths from other causes. Emerson and Braverman (1980) have cited reports dating back to 1949 on the use of x-rays on the heads and necks of children for the treatment of such conditions as thymic enlargement, tinea capitis, benign hemangiomas, and whooping cough, as well as the use of ^{131}I for hyperthyroidism. All of these cases reveal an abnormally high incidence of benign and malignant thyroid tumors. In another study (Baverstock, Papworth, & Vennart, 1981) of 110 women who also worked with paint containing radium between 1939 and 1971, and in whom exposure was not greatly in excess of current recommendations of the International Commission on Radiation Protection (ICRP), there was a highly significant excess of breast cancer.

Two further discoveries in the 1930s added to the nature and magnitude of the radiation hazards already presented by x-rays and radium, as well as contributing potentially significant benefits. The first was the discovery by the Joliot-Curies that any element can be made radioactive, as, for example, when alpha particles emitted by plutonium strike an aluminum plate and the aluminum continues to give off electrons long after the plutonium source has been removed. This discovery heralded the beginning of the extensive use of artificially produced radioactive isotopes. The second was the splitting of the atom by Hahn and Strassman during the course of bombarding uranium with neutrons. This led to the discovery that a mass of uranium can undergo a sequence of nuclear fissions (a chain reaction) and to the development of nuclear weapons for waging war and nuclear power plants as a source of energy.

The principal activities since World War II that constitute important sources of human radiation exposure are (1) the medical uses of x-rays and radioactive isotopes, (2) uranium mining, (3) radioactive fallout from the atmospheric detonation of nuclear weapons, (4) radioactive elements deriving from the operation of nuclear power plants, and (5) the disposal of radioactive wastes.

In 1947, Mole already thought that it was "probably true to say that more is known about the biological effects of radiation than of any other environmental hazard except bacteria" (cited in Van Cleave, 1968). Indeed, the first two decades of the use of x-rays and radium provided ample evidence that these agents can cause eye irritation, cataracts, dermatitis, hair loss, and cancerous ulcers. Early studies on animals also showed an inhibition of bone growth as well as abnormalities of bone growth and the development of sterility.

Other effects of radiation recorded later include cell killing, the induction of genetic defects and cancer, life-span shortening, and the impairment of immune function. Nevertheless, it is evident from the BEIR III Report (1980, pp. 261–264) that many controversial issues remain regarding the effects of exposure to low levels of ionizing radiation on human populations.

Virtually all of the disorders attributable to radiation exposure also can develop "spontaneously," and it therefore becomes necessary to show, generally by epidemiologic methods, that a suspected radiation-induced disorder indeed represents a significantly increased incidence. Except for those rare instances in which there is an isolated exposure of a definitive group, as in the case of the luminizers or the uranium miners, what often makes such proof difficult is that there is a characteristically long latent period between exposure and the appearance of an induced disorder, during which time many of the exposed individuals move and cannot be traced.

TYPES OF RADIOACTIVITY AND THEIR UNITS OF MEASUREMENT

Radiation can be defined as one of a number of processes by which energy is emitted and transferred; it can be ionizing or nonionizing. Ionizing radiation includes alpha, beta, or gamma rays; x-rays; electrons; neutrons; and cosmic rays. Van Cleave (1968) defines ionization as

> . . . the process by which a fast moving quantity of energy, striking an atom or molecule, transfers all or part of its energy to the atom and leaves it in an electrically disturbed or charged state. The production of charged particles, or ions, is mainly responsible for initiating the physicochemical changes in living cells which lead ultimately to the production of overt radiation damage. The physical effects of ionization are over in a fraction of a second, but the biological effects of the disrupted molecule may not appear for hours, days, months or even years.

Nonionizing radiation passes through or strikes matter without transferring its energy and produces no effect. Visible light, infrared, and some ultraviolet radiations do not produce ionization in living matter.

The biological effect of a given type of radiation depends on the energy absorbed in a cell or tissue. Ionizing radiations, although they have a common effect on living matter, differ in their origin and physical properties. X-rays and gamma rays are electromagnetic waves like visible light, while the other ionizing radiations just noted consist of streams of individual particles. Alpha, beta, gamma, and sometimes other radiations are emitted during the disintegration of unstable (radioactive) atomic nuclei. One or more such disintegrations can convert the unstable nucleus into a stable one; for example, radium ultimately transforms into stable lead. Table 4–1 compares the penetrating power of the biologically important types of ionizing radiation.

The *radioactive half-life* is defined as the time required for a radioactive isotope to lose 50 percent of its activity in this decay process. Table 4-2 provides some perspective on the range of half-lives of isotopes.

X-rays and gamma rays, on the other hand, are electromagnetic waves with similar biological effects. Radioisotopes are common sources of gamma rays. X-rays usually are produced by electrons striking the anode of an x-ray tube. The penetrating power of x-rays is determined by the magnitude of the electron-accelerating voltage applied to the tube. The x-rays used for diagnostic medical procedures are less energetic and less penetrating than gamma rays from any radioisotope.

The radiation energy dose absorbed by any material is measured in rads. One rad is equal to an energy absorption of 100 ergs/gm of irradiated matter. The roentgen (R) is the unit in which exposures to x- or gamma rays are often expressed. It is defined and measured in terms of the ionization produced in air under specific conditions, and it cannot be applied to radiation other than x- and gamma rays. The rem (roentgen equivalent man) is a dose unit that equals the dose in rads times the appropriate value of relative biological effectiveness (RBE) for the particular radiation (rads × RBE = rems). Thus, rad and roentgen are physical measurements of energy, while rem takes into account the type of radiation and the magnitude of effect this radiation will have on a given biological system.

Table 4-1 Comparison of Penetrating Power of Biologically Important Types of Ionizing Radiation

Type	Composition	Source	Order of Magnitude of Range in Tissue (cm)
Alpha rays	Helium nuclei	Certain radioactive heavy isotopes	0.005
Beta rays	Electrons	Radioisotopes	0.1
Gamma rays	Electromagnetic radiation	Radioisotopes	10.0
X-rays	Electromagnetic radiation	X-ray machines	10.0
Cosmic rays	Electrons, mesons, x- and gamma rays	Radiation from outer space produces secondary radiation in the atmosphere	100.0

Source: Data from A. M. Brues (ed.). *Low-Level Irradiation.* Washington, D.C.: American Association for the Advancement of Science, 1959.

Table 4-2   Radioactive Half-Life
of Some Isotopes

Isotope	Radioactive Half-Life
Potassium-42	12.4 hrs
Sodium-24	14.9 hrs
Bromium-82	35.0 hrs
Gold-198	2.7 days
Iodine-131	8.1 days
Phosphorus-32	14.3 days
Iodine-125	60.0 days
Tantalum-182	111.0 days
Cobalt-60	5.3 yrs
Tritium (H-3)	12.3 yrs
Strontium-90	28.0 yrs
Cesium-137	33.0 yrs
Radium-37	1600.0 yrs
Carbon-14	5730.0 yrs

The distribution of dose with regard to time is also an important consideration. Either the total dose over a delineated period or the dose delivered per unit time (dose rate) may be used. A protracted irradiation at a low dose rate usually is considered to be a long-term exposure. Short-term exposure includes total body exposure over a short time, as in nuclear warfare; as well as limited body exposure, as in therapeutic or diagnostic radiology. When the irradiation is interrupted rather than continuous, it is referred to as a fractionnated dose.

In evaluating the potential harm of a radioactive isotope that is ingested or otherwise absorbed by the body, there are several factors to consider in addition to the radioactive half-life, which is an indicator of the potential duration of irradiation. The distribution of isotopes within the body is also a consideration. Some isotopes such as sodium and potassium (or cesium, which is distributed like potassium) are disseminated widely as electrolytes. Others such as calcium and iodine have distinct target sites. For calcium (and also for strontium, which is distributed like calcium), the target sites are bone and teeth, while the target organ for iodine isotopes is the thyroid. Thus certain isotopes may create "hot spots" of radioactivity by virtue of their concentration in particular organs. Another factor is the *biological half-life* which is defined as the time required for the body to eliminate half an administered dose of any substance by regular processes of elimination. The *effective half-life*, which is defined as the time required for a radioactive element in the body to be diminished by one half, can be calculated from the following formula:

$$\text{Effective half-life} = \frac{(\text{Biological half-life})(\text{Radioactive half-life})}{\text{Biological half-life} + \text{Radioactive half-life}}$$

SOURCES OF HUMAN EXPOSURE

The BEIR III Report (1980) lists the four principal categories of radiation exposure. These include natural background radiation, radiation in the healing arts, environmental radiation deriving from the production and use of nuclear energy, and a miscellaneous category.

Natural Background Radiation

The BEIR III Report (1980), among others, states that "natural background remains the greatest contributor to the radiation exposure of the U. S. population today" (p. 37). Perhaps the repetition of such statements is intended to assure the public that small additions to this basal burden are unlikely to be harmful.

Background radiation has three components: (1) terrestrial radiation, (2) cosmic radiation arising from outer space, and (3) naturally occurring radionuclides. Exposure to terrestrial radiation varies with geographic location and living habits. The dose-equivalent (DE) rate, which is a measure of the effective absorbed dose, varies with the type of soil in a given area and its naturally occurring radionuclides. The conterminous United States can be divided into three broad areas in respect to DE rates, as shown in Table 4–3.

Cosmic radiation includes both the particles of extraterrestrial origin that penetrate the earth's atmosphere and the particles generated when these primary particles strike the atmosphere. The earth's

Table 4-3 Comparison by Area of Range of Exposure to
Terrestrial Radiation

Area	Rate of Dose Equivalent (DE)*
Atlantic and Gulf Coastal Plain	15–35 mrem/yr (avg 23 mrem)
Northeastern, Central, and Far Western Areas	35–75 mrem/yr (avg 46 mrem)
Colorado Plateau Area	75–140 mrem/yr (avg 90 mrem)

*The average DE rate to the U.S. population from terrestrial sources (disregarding structural shielding) is estimated to be about 40 mrem/yr.

Source: Data from BEIR III Report (Committee on the Biological Effects of Ionizing Radiations). *The Effects on Populations of Exposure to Low Levels of Ionizing Radiation*. Washington, D.C.: National Academy Press, 1980.

atmosphere serves as a shield against cosmic radiation, so the thinner the shield the greater the DE rate. Thinning of this shield by commercial products such as the fluorocarbon propellants in spray cans is therefore a matter of public concern. The DE rate for cosmic radiation increases with altitude (at 1800 meters it is double that at sea level), and it also varies with changes in the earth's magnetic field. The DE rate also varies owing to solar modulation. The average DE rate to the U.S. population from cosmic radiation is estimated to be about 31 mrem/yr.

The effects of naturally occurring radionuclides, unlike terrestrial and cosmic radiation, are internal, resulting from inhalation and ingestion of these materials in air, food, and water. These radioactive elements include lead, polonium, bismuth, radium, radon, potassium, carbon, hydrogen, uranium, thorium, and others. Radioactivity from this source has been measured in the gonads, lungs, gastrointestinal tract, bone cortex, and bone marrow.

Radiation in the Healing Arts

Studies carried out by the Bureau of Radiological Health (BRH) between 1973 and 1977, and cited in the BEIR III Report (1980), show that the largest source of radiation exposure of the U.S. population to human-made radiation is from the use of x-rays. The BRH report estimates that over 300,000 x-ray units were being used for medical diagnosis and therapy—about 170,000 by dentists and about 130,000 by physicians, chiropractors, and podiatrists. A small number of additional units still were being used in vans for chest x-rays.

The BRH studies also estimate that about 129 million people (about two-thirds of the U.S. population) have been exposed to medical and dental x-rays. Table 4–4 summarizes information on per capita bone marrow exposure from these x-ray examinations. The correlation of age with increasing exposure reflects the preponderant use of medical services by the elderly. The Environmental Protection Agency (EPA) has estimated that people who work with x-ray equipment in medicine and dentistry received an average DE of about 50 mrem in 1975.

Over 10,000 physicians in the United States are licensed to administer radiopharmaceuticals, and it has been estimated that some 10 to 12 million doses are administered annually. About 90 percent of the reported procedures involved seven organ systems. Listed in order of frequency, they are brain, liver, bone, lung, thyroid, kidney,

Table 4–4   Per Capita Mean Active Bone Marrow Dose for Specific Age Groups from Medical X-ray Procedures in 1970

Age	Per Capita Mean Active Bone Marrow Dose (mrad)
15–24	52
25–34	81
35–44	107
45–54	120
55–64	143
65 and over	151

Source: B. Shleien, T. T. Tucker, and D. W. Johnson. *The Mean Active Bone Marrow Dose in the Adult Population of the United States from Diagnostic Radiology*. Rockville, Md.: USDHEW, 1977, FDA publication no. 77-8013.

and heart. The age distribution of patient exposure to radionuclides is similar to that for x-ray exposure.

The EPA also has estimated that whole-body patient doses from the diagnostic use of radiopharmaceuticals represent about 20 percent of the patient doses resulting from medical diagnostic radiology. In addition, the EPA has estimated that the 80,000 or more people who work with radionuclides and radium receive a mean annual dose of 260 mrem from the radionuclides and 540 mrem from radium.

Radiation from the Production and Use of Nuclear Energy

During the 1950s and 1960s, when extensive testing of nuclear devices was conducted in the atmosphere, large quantities of radioactive materials were released into the atmosphere, disseminated throughout the world by the prevailing winds, and deposited on the earth's surface with rainfall. The dose received from fallout varied with the distance from the site of the explosion. Probably the first public awareness of this phenomenon derived from news media reports of exposure to fallout by two groups of people downwind from an explosion in the Bikini Atoll on March 1, 1954. Those most severely irradiated were 23 Japanese fishermen aboard the small trawler Lucky Dragon Number 5, and 239 natives on the tiny islands of Rongelap, Ailinginae, and Uterik, as well as 28 Americans on Rongerik.

Two weeks after this explosion, radioactivity measures of various areas of the Lucky Dragon were as high as 50 to 150 milliroentgens per hour, and it was generally believed that the fishermen must have received about 200 roentgens of total body radiation. Shortly after the Lucky Dragon incident, the tuna from it delivered to an Osaka market showed counts of 10,000 per minute on a Geiger counter (natural background is 30 to 40 counts per minute). The Japanese then monitored fish arriving at this market for six more weeks, checking 564 fishing boats. Some 213,000 pounds of contaminated fish were confiscated.

The Lucky Dragon incident is illustrative of potential effects outside the delineated danger area for acute radiation injury. In addition, radionuclides deposited with rainfall can enter the food chain.

When they are deposited in the water they may enter the tissues of aquatic animals consumed by humans, or they may enter human tissues more directly via the drinking water. The radionuclides deposited in the soil may be absorbed by the root systems of plants that humans eat or use as animal feed. In the latter case, humans may consume radioactive meat and dairy products. During the 1950s and 1960s there were excessive levels of radioactivity in food and dairy products throughout the United States, deriving from atmospheric tests carried out in the Nevada desert.

Although much of the radionuclide debris has decayed since the tests of 20 to 30 years ago, the small amount that remains from isotopes with long half-lives will continue to be a source of exposure to the United States population for some years. In addition, there are still occasional atmospheric tests by countries in the early stages of developing atomic weapons. The BEIR III Report (1980, p. 53) sums up the 50-year dose commitment in the North Temperate zone from nuclear tests concluded by 1971 as follows: gonads — 170 mrem; bone lining cells — 260 mrem; bone marrow — 230 mrem. It also projects annual whole-body DE to the United States population from previous atmospheric tests as falling from 13 mrem, the 1963 level, to 4.9 mrem in the year 2000.

According to the BEIR III Report (1980), as of April 1979, 70 nuclear power reactors had been licensed for operation in the United States. An additional 73 nonpower nuclear reactors were in use for tests, research, and university applications; about 80 were being operated by the Department of Energy (DOE); and 174 were in operation or under construction by the military. The number of additional reactors to be built in future years is presently in considerable doubt, largely as a consequence of public reaction to the Three Mile Island accident and because the economy of nuclear reactors as a source of energy is being questioned as the costs of construction, operation, and clean-up of accidents escalate.

A variety of activities support reactor operations. One of these is the mining and milling of uranium. According to the BEIR III Report (1980), there are several hundred uranium mines in operation, employing about 5000 people. There are also 20 uranium mills and 21 fuel fabrication plants in operation. The report states that there have been problems with radionuclide release from uranium mills, but it does not detail the nature of these problems. The disposal of tailings from uranium mines also has been a matter of concern among residents in the vicinity of the mines. The storage of spent fuel and the disposal of radioactive wastes, as well as the reprocessing of fuels remain serious unsolved and controversial problems (see Chapter 7).

In addition to the risks that confront workers associated with nuclear power reactors, there also are risks to the general population. Included among the latter are populations in the vicinity in which radioactive wastes are stored. There are risks from nuclear power accidents, as well as from the routine operation of nuclear power plants. The radionuclides of particular concern in the event of a major reactor accident are strontium-90 and cesium-17. Three radionuclides of significance in respect to the routine operation of nuclear power plants are tritium (hydrogen-3), carbon-14, and krypton-85, all of which are discharged daily and continuously into adjacent streams or rivers in the coolant water. These are difficult to remove or confine. The problem that they pose is comparable to that from fallout in that they may contaminate drinking water as well as fish; they also may enter the food chain if the contaminated streams or rivers are used for the irrigation of crops for animal fodder or crops for human consumption. Particularly noteworthy in this regard is tritium, which is readily incorporated into the DNA of cells (Dobson & Cooper, 1974; Dobson & Kwan, 1976), the significance of which is discussed in the following section.

Miscellaneous Sources of Radiation

Several products yield ionizing radiation or contain radioactive materials. Included among the latter are television sets, luminous-dial watches, luggage x-ray inspection systems at airports, dental prostheses, smoke detectors, high-voltage vacuum switches, electron microscopes, static eliminators, cardiac pacemakers, tobacco products, fossil fuels, and certain building materials. Another source of irradiation exposure is from cosmic radiation during air flight, as well as from the shipment of radioactive materials by commercial aircraft. The estimated DE rate for the United States population from radioactive materials in products is estimated to be four to five mrem/yr, and from travel in commerical aircraft about 3.1 mrem/yr.

However, the estimated exposure of cabin attendants and aircraft crew is 160 mrem/yr.

Summary

Table 4-5 summarizes radiation exposure from the various sources discussed above. It would appear that, despite statements to the contrary already noted, exposure from human-made sources is now greater, on the average, than from natural background radiation.

This use of averages may appear reassuring, but like all averages there are locations and situations where exposures are higher and others where they are lower. Moreover, they do not reflect occupational exposures and other special situations such as the disposal of mine tailings in the vicinity of uranium mines. They also do not reflect radiation related to the disposal of radioactive wastes. In 1979, about 80,000 cubic meters of low-level waste were buried in the United States, a volume equivalent to about 366,000 55-gallon drums, each with about 200 microcuries of activity (Casarett, 1981) (see Chapter 7). Nor do the averages listed in Table 4-5 reflect the

Table 4-5   Summary of Sources of Exposure to Irradiation of the General Population[a]

Sources	Average Exposure mrem/yr
Natural background	80.0
Medical and dental x-rays	78.4
Radiopharmaceuticals	13.6
Atmospheric nuclear weapons tests	4.5
Commercial nuclear power plants	1.0
Consumer products and miscellaneous	4.5

[a]General population denotes people of all ages except those whose work is radiation related or commonly exposes them to extra radiation.
Source: Data from BEIR III Report (Committee on the Biological Effects of Ionizing Radiation). *The Effects on Populations of Exposure to Low Levels of Ionizing Radiation*. Washington, D.C.: National Academy Press, 1980, pp. 66–67.

fact that certain relatively long-lived isotopes have a predilection for certain tissues or structures where exposure may therefore be of long duration. Finally, if the average exposure of less than one mrem/yr from commercial nuclear power plants was determined by dividing total environmental radiation from this source by the United States population, it would not reflect exposure in the vicinity of the plants. There are radiobiologists like Lindop (1981) who believe that "the radiation to the population may prove to be the factor limiting the use of nuclear energy."

THE MANIFESTATIONS OF
IRRADIATION DAMAGE

While it generally is assumed that radiation damage has its origin in individual cells, there is a diversity of cell types and arrangements in forming organs; these may influence the probability of radiation damage. Organs possess supporting connective tissue that may provide a shield for cellular components. The blood supply and nerves also course within this supporting structure. Moreover, cell types vary in respect to their sensitivity. There are cells that undergo division on a regular cyclic schedule, such as the epidermis of the skin and the epithelium of the intestinal tract. Cells of this type with a high rate of turnover are generally radiosensitive. Other types of cells undergo division on a demand basis and thereby maintain an equilibrium. Germ cells and cells of the hemopoietic system are examples of this type, and they also are radiosensitive, particularly when in a state of rapid cell division. Finally, there are cells that lose their capacity for further division shortly after birth. The neurons of the brain, heart muscle cells, and certain types of kidney cells are examples of this type, and they are relatively radioresistant; however, when killed, they are not replaced.

Damage to cells can occur as a result of direct hits by ionizing irradiation, but damage also can occur indirectly. One of the relatively late effects of irradiation is the formation of interstitial scar tissue. Whether this results from radiation damage of blood vessels or as a direct consequence of the radiation is uncertain, but the ultimate result is an impairment of blood supply and deprivation of cells of oxygen and nutrients, as well as of the channels through which cells discharge waste products.

Effects of Irradiation on Cells

When an organism is irradiated, there are four possible consequences: (1) the radiation may pass through the body without striking any cells; (2) some part of a cell may be hit and the damage repaired; (3) the cell may be damaged in such a way that it cannot reproduce itself, or it may be destroyed; or (4) the cell may be damaged and survive to produce a clone of perturbated cells.

The extreme effect is cell killing. At high radiation doses, when a large number of cells are killed, recovery of organ function depends upon the ability of stem cells to replace those that are destroyed. At low levels of irradiation there may be no detectable interference with normal function, since the relatively small number of cells killed is replaced rapidly. An exception is irradiation of cells of the developing fetus, since during organogenesis the destruction of only a few cells can interfere with proper organ development and there may be teratogenic effects.

Another important effect of irradiation of cells is the suppression of cell division—radiation-induced mitotic arrest. It is common to encounter multinucleated forms in irradiated cells in tissue culture.

An important type of radiation-induced cell perturbation is mutation. Mutated somatic cells that survive may give rise to cancer, immunodeficiency disorders, or accelerated aging. On the other hand, mutations of germ cells that survive may give rise later to genetic effects. These are discussed later in this section. Mutations arise as a result of damage to DNA by ionizing radiation.

The visible structural effect of the irradiation of cells is the damaging of chromosomes. This may include fragmentation of chromosomes, exchanges of segments between chromosomes, development of abnormal forms such as ring and dicentric forms (Figure 4-1), and a reduction or an increase in the number of chromosomes.

Genetic and Congenital Effects of Irradiation

Genetic disorders, by definition, do not occur in persons whose germ cells have been affected by radiation; the effects are seen in their offspring and in later generations to which the altered genetic material is transmitted. Genetic disorders caused by radiation ex-

Figure 4-1 Cells Showing Chromosome Abnormalities following X-irradiation (arrows indicate a dicentric form in the upper figure and a ring form in the lower figure).

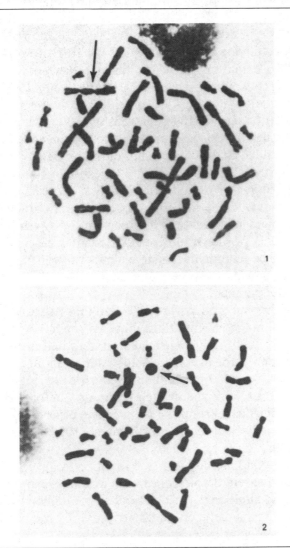

Source: T. Ishihara and T. Kumatori. Chromosome Studies on Japanese Exposed to Radiation Resulting from Nuclear Bomb Explosion. In H. J. Evans, W. M. Court Brown, and A. S. McLean (eds.), *Human Radiation Cytogenetics*. Amsterdam, Netherlands: North-Holland Publishing Co., 1967, p. 128. Used with permission.

posure result either from changes in individual genes or changes in chromosomes. On the other hand, congenital effects are those observed in the offspring following maternal irradiation during gestation.

Prior to World War II, "ionizing radiation was simply a laboratory tool for studying genetic principles" (BEIR III Report, 1980, p. 72). In 1956, a committee of the National Academy of Sciences/National Research Council was set up to study "the biological effects of atomic radiation" (the BEAR Committee). Using an average background radiation level of five roentgens over 30 years and a radiation level from medical exposure of three roentgens, this committee recommended that human-made radiation be so limited as to keep the average individual exposure to less than 10 roentgens before the mean age of reproduction, that is, 30 years. Employing laboratory animal data, the BEIR III study used two models to estimate the changes in incidence of disorders caused by gene mutations: (1) the incidence of such disorders expected after the continuous exposure of the population over a large number of generations (2) the incidence of disorders expected in a single generation after the exposure of the parents.

By the first method, it was estimated that only one to six percent of all spontaneous mutations that occur in humans can be ascribed to the effects of average background radiation. An increase in exposure above the average would result in an increased mutation rate of 60 to 1100 per million liveborn offspring per rem of parental exposure received in each generation before conception. The current incidence (resulting from causes other than radiation) of human genetic disorders is approximately 107,000 cases per million liveborns.

In the second method of risk estimation, an average parental exposure of one rem before conception would be expected to produce five to 65 additional genetic disorders per million liveborn offspring. Significantly, the estimates arrived at by the two different methods are in good agreement.

Disorders due to chromosomal aberrations—estimated from the chromosomal aberration incidence seen in a late developmental stage of spermatocytes and made with the assumption that the risk for oocytes is of equal size—come to fewer than 10 anomalies per million liveborn. However, numerous studies have shown a high incidence of chromosomal aberrations in spontaneously aborted human embryos and fetuses, and evidently no attempt has been made to relate these to either natural background or human-made radiation. It may be that an estimate of radiation-induced abortions associated with chromosomal aberrations is also not possible. Abnormalities of autosomal chromosomes appear to have such a devastating effect on blastogenesis that the conceptus implants briefly or not at all—a so-called "occult abortion." This takes place within two weeks after ovulation, before there may even be an awareness of pregnancy.

The effects of irradiation damage to sperm or ova and of maternal uterine irradiation during pregnancy may be quite similar. Maternal irradiation early in pregnancy may lead to death and expulsion of the embryo. If irradiation occurs during major organogenesis, major malformations commonly occur. General growth retardation, either temporary or permanent, also may occur. Irradiation during the fetal period also can produce localized growth retardation and effects on germ-cell populations and the central nervous system. Some of these may be present at birth, while others (fertility depression, lifespan shortening, neuronal depletion) may find expression later.

Abnormalities that have been reported after *in utero* irradiation include microcephaly, mental retardation, growth retardation, hydrocephaly, microphthalmia, coloboma, chorioretinitis, blindness, strabismus, nystagmus, coordination defects, mongolism, spina bifida, skull malformations, cleft palate, ear abnormalities, deformed hands, clubfeet, hypophalangism, and genital deformities (BEIR III Report, 1980).

Radiological Carcinogenesis

Of all of the abnormalities resulting from irradiation, cancer induction clearly has received the greatest attention. Nevertheless, much remains controversial regarding carcinogenesis following low-dose ionizing irradiation. There are convincing data that cancer induction occurs in humans over a range of high doses, but at doses of only a few rads the evidence is statistical and often cannot be attributed with certainty to radiation. Estimation of cancer risk at low doses usually involves extrapolation from observations at higher doses on the basis of assumptions about the nature of the dose-response relationship, as discussed later.

Cancers induced by radiation are indistinguishable from those associated with other causes, and the indication that radiation may be causal can be inferred only on the basis of a statistical excess above the natural incidence. Cancer can be induced by radiation in almost all of the tissues of the human body, although tissues and organs vary considerably in their sensitivity to such induction. The natural incidence of cancer involves several variables that also must be taken into account in assessing radiation as causal; these include the type and site of origin of the neoplasm, age and sex of the patient, and other factors.

While solid tumors are greater numerically than leukemia following whole-body exposure, they characteristically have long latent periods (10 to 30 years after radiation), whereas the excess cases of leukemia appear within a few years after exposure. The major sites of radiation-induced solid cancers in women are the breast and the thyroid gland. For solid tumors at other sites of origin, the risks in the two sexes are approximately equal.

Age at exposure is an important variable in the risk of cancer. The clearest evidence for an age factor is the very high risk of leukemia in those irradiated during the first year of life; the evidence for this first emerged among atomic bomb survivors. In adults there is a rising excess of risk of leukemia with increasing age. The evidence for this emerged from studies in the United Kingdom on patients irradiated for ankylosing spondylitis (Court Brown & Doll, 1965), as well as from atomic bomb survivors in Japan (Bizzozero, Johnson, & Ciocco, 1966), despite the difference in the incidence of spontaneous leukemia in the two countries. With respect to solid tumors, women exposed in the second decade of life, when major hormonal changes are taking place, appear to be at highest risk for breast cancer. Generally, solid tumors show a longer latent period in younger subjects than in older ones, in contrast to leukemia in which there are shorter appearance times in children than in adults.

A variety of host and environmental factors complicates the evaluation of dose–response relationships. Among these are hormonal influences, cell stimulators, immunological status, exposure to other oncogenic agents, and the state of DNA repair mechanisms.

The increase in free radicals in cells following irradiation is particularly important in carcinogenesis. These free radicals are believed to represent the ultimate agent that attacks DNA and thereby causes carcinogenic transformation. However, radiation also may cause cancer indirectly by permitting the expression of the carcinogenic potential of a passenger virus. The evidence for this comes largely from animal studies. This effect requires relatively high doses of radiation. Experimental data support the possibility that radiation causes cancer at any dose by direct attack on cellular DNA via free radicals, while at high doses it may sometimes involve the action of oncogenic viruses.

The variety of possible biological mechanisms responsibile for human cancer in general suggests that the dose–response relationships may vary for different types of radiation-induced cancer. In addition, the dose–incidence relationship for internally deposited radionuclides may be different than for external body irradiation, because of marked nonuniformities in the distribution of radiation in the body. Finally, a distinction should be made between cancer incidence and cancer mortality. Some skin and some thyroid cancers do not greatly alter the death rate, whereas leukemia and lung and breast cancer have high mortality rates.

Radiation and Aging

The conditions under which irradiation may be regarded as responsible for premature aging have been summed up in the BEIR III Report (1980, p. 501) as follows:

Radiation causes the force of mortality to increase more rapidly in exposed than in unexposed subjects without altering the shape of the cumulative mortality curve.

Exposure results in a proportionate decrease in the age of onset of all diseases or causes of death that affect the control group without altering the degree, sequence, or absolute incidence of the diseases and causes of death.

Radiation causes all the morphologic and physiologic manifestations of the aging process to appear and develop at proportionately earlier chronological ages, to degrees and rates in the various organs proportional to the degrees and rates in organs of unexposed subjects.

An important issue in gerontology is the relationship of biological aging to those diseases that increase in prevalence with advancing age. The development of concepts that consider this issue is therefore relevant to this discussion. These concepts were proposed first by Failla (1958), Curtis and Gebhard (1958), and Szilard (1959). It is noteworthy that the first two were radiobiologists and the third a nuclear physicist. They proposed that spontaneous mutations of somatic cells accumulate randomly over time, and they drew an analogy between this phenomenon and "hits" resulting from irradiation. These cells then function differently from the original population of cells and may account for the progressive loss of organ function associated with aging.

Curtis (1966) discovered that there is a steady increase in chromosome aberrations with age in mouse liver cells, an observation similar to that reported in studies on human lymphocytes (Jacobs, Court Brown, & Doll, 1961). Curtis also found that, following a single x-ray dose large enough to shorten life expectancy, there was a sudden increase in chromosome aberrations, which decreased slowly over a period of many months. The degree of life shortening was quantitatively related to the amount of chromosome damage. In studying inbred mice with different lifespans, Curtis discovered that the stability of chromosomes as indicated by radiation sensitivity is inversely related to longevity. Moreover, the irradiated mice show striking external evidence of premature aging.

These earlier studies on mutation theory have been expanded to include a broader concept designated "error catastrophe concept" (Burnet, 1983), which holds that over time there is an accumulation of DNA replication errors leading to a progressive accumulation of misspecified structural, hormonal, enzymal, and antibody proteins. A substantial body of evidence, particularly regarding the identification of misspecified enzymes, has been reported in the gerontology literature. Misspecification of proteins not only may account for the progressive decline in physiological function but also may constitute both direct and indirect factors in the genesis of those diseases prevalent in old age, including cancer, arteriosclerosis (Benditt & Benditt, 1973) and diabetes (Gabbay, 1980; Rotwein, Chyn, & Chirgwin, 1981).

Aside from the possibility that misspecification of proteins may be a direct cause of disease, it also may account for the aging-related loss of DNA repair capacity, as well as the loss of immune competency. In their normal state, DNA repair and immune responses may serve as natural protection against radiation damage. While little is known about the effect of total-body irradiation on DNA repair capacity, both aging and irradiation result in a reduction in immune competency and the appearance of autoimmune disease, as discussed in the following section.

It is noteworthy in respect to the foregoing that, as early as 1956, Warren reported a retrospective study on the lifespan of over 80,000 physicians varying in respect to their exposure to radiation. As shown in Table 4–6, there is about a three- to five-year reduction in the lifespan of radiologists as compared with other physicians; and while many radiologists died of leukemia, practically every other cause of death also was represented, including cardiovascular-renal disease. These observations were confirmed later by Seltser and Sartwell (1965) and Matanoski, Seltser, Sartwell, et al., (1975a,b), as well as by Radford et al. (1977) in a comparison of irradiated and nonirradiated ankylosing spondylitis patients. While these more recent studies have shown a diminution in deaths from leukemia, this disease has been replaced by lymphoma and multiple myeloma. Moreover, the previously cited study on irradiated peptic ulcer patients (Peters et al., 1980) also showed earlier mortalities not only from cancer but from other causes as well.

Nevertheless, the BEIR III Report (1980) concluded that "ionizing radiation induces or accelerates some but not all diseases, de-

Table 4–6 Effect of Radiation on the Lifespan of Physicians

Category	Average Lifespan
No known contact with radiation	65.7
Some exposure (dermatologists, gastroenterologists, urologists, tuberculosis specialists)	63.3
Radiologists	60.5
U.S. population over 20 years of age	67.1

Source: Data from S. Warren. Longevity and Causes of Death from Irradiation in Physicians. *JAMA*, 1956, *162*:464–468.

pending on the genetic susceptibility of the subject and the exposure conditions. For doses of less than approximately 300 rads of low LET (linear energy transfer) radiation, the principal mechanism of life-shortening is the induction or acceleration of neoplastic diseases."

The areas of aging in which radiation shows little or no accelerating effect are those involving biochemical and physiological changes that are not life threatening. These include alterations in collagen, pigment accumulation, neuromuscular function, and the like. As with aging, however, radiation exposure does result in an increase in interstitial fibrosis of a variety of organs and increased arteriocapillary fibrosis. However, it is not known whether the mechanism that produces these changes is, in each instance, the same as that in natural aging. Radiation also produces cataracts, and, while age-dependent factors may be involved in this effect, it is not known if the mechanism is similar to senescent cataract formation.

Radiation and the Immune System

As already noted, there are mechanisms that retard or prevent both carcinogenesis and aging. Principally these are DNA repair systems and immune phenomena. While radiation and other mutagenic agents have been used as tools for identifying DNA repair mechanisms, the effect of radiation on DNA repair itself evidently has not been investigated. Yet such an effect appears quite likely, since DNA repair involves excision and replacement of DNA segments, a process facilitated by enzyme proteins themselves specified by DNA. On the other hand, the effects of aging and of irradiation on the immune system have been studied and a comparison of these two is relevant here.

Weksler (1981) comments that we appear to be approaching a unitary immunologic theory of aging in which a genetically programmed age-associated disorder of immunoregulation may account for not only chronic low-grade tissue damage but also for the rising incidence of neoplastic disease, infections, autoimmunity, and atherosclerotic vascular disease. The autoimmunity may account not only for some direct tissue destruction but also for a variety of immune-complex disorders, including senile amyloidosis.

There is surprisingly little coverage of radiation effects on the immune system in publications dealing primarily in radiobiology; for example the BEIR III Report (1980) makes scant mention of radiation-induced immunodeficiency disorders. Older studies show that irradiation produces a decline in the capacity to synthesize humoral antibody and to mount an anamnestic response to a secondary introduction of antigen (Van Cleave, 1968). These effects are comparable to the aging-related decline in humoral antibody response noted previously. There also are more recent studies that deal with the effects of irradiation on T-lymphocyte activities. At low doses (five to 25 rads), *in vitro* studies reveal an augmentation of the immune response (Anderson & Lefkovits, 1979) that is attributed to injury to an exquisitely radiosensitive subpopulation of suppressor T cells, again an effect similar to that associated with aging. There is also evidence deriving from a comparison of irradiated thymectomized and shamthymectomized mice suggesting that some of the carcinogenic and life-shortening effects of irradiation may be mediated by T-cell injury (Anderson et al., 1980). The latter report draws an analogy between the effects of thymectomy and radiation in respect to lifespan shortening, cancer, and autoimmunity. Other studies indicate an acceleration of amyloidosis following irradiation (Lesher, Grahn, & Sallese, 1957; Kellum, Sutherland, Eckert, et al., 1965; Janigan & Druet, 1968; Musacchia & Blumenthal, in press).

Dose–Response Relationships

The atomic bombs dropped on Japan near the end of World War II and the atmospheric nuclear weapons tests of the following two decades served to arouse widespread public concern regarding harmful effects of ionizing radiation, even at low levels. This concern was reflected in the initiation of measurements of natural background radiation and in acceptance of the concept of regulating overall population exposure. As previously noted, the NAS/NRC BEAR (Biological Effects of Atomic Radiation) Committee recommended that average individual exposure from radiation other than background be limited to no more than 10 roentgens between conception and age 30, that is, the reproductive period. Around the same time, another body, the National Council on Radiation Protection

(BEIR III, 1980) recommended that the permissible dose to the general population from other than medical and dental sources be no larger than that due to natural background. Radiation Protection Guides are stated in rems rather than roentgens (R) to take into account biological effectiveness and its dependence on radiation quality. Thus, the BEAR Committee divided the 10-rem recommended ceiling into five rems from medical procedures and five rems from nonmedical sources.

Morgan (1978) points out that there have been several subsequent reductions in the permissible exposure levels for both occupational workers and for the public. The occupational maximum permissible exposure level has dropped by a factor of 10 and the level for the public by a factor of 300. This dual standard makes it evident that considerations other than scientific data enter into these decisions. Morgan (1979–1980) argues that "national and international setting bodies and many who are strongly pronuclear accept the studies which support the lower risk estimates as though their accuracy and certainty were validated by Divine decree while they severely criticize and refuse to make use of the findings from the studies that show a high cancer risk from low level radiation exposure" (p. 2). Table 4–7 provides a list of bodies that have had a role in decisions affecting the exposure to radioactivity.

What lends support to Morgan's argument are reports of an excessive risk of cancer and other radiation-related disorders in situations where exposure is carefully monitored to make certain that the maximum permissible exposure is not exceeded. Already noted in

Table 4-7   A List of Bodies with a Nuclear Regulatory Role

National Council on Radiation Protection (NCRP)
Atomic Energy Commission (AEC); now Department of Energy (DOE)
Federal Radiation Council (FRC)
International Commission on Radiological Protection (ICRP)
Environmental Protection Agency (EPA)
Bureau of Radiological Health (BRH)
Nuclear Regulatory Commission (NRC)
Committee on the Biological Effects of Ionizing Radiation (BEIR)
United Nations Scientific Committee on the Effects of Atomic Radiation
   (UNSCEAR)

this regard is the increased incidence of leukemia and multiple myeloma as well as a decrease in lifespan from cancer and other age-related diseases among radiologists. Furthermore, Mancuso, Stewart, and Kneale (1977) found a higher-than-expected rate of multiple myeloma among radiation workers at the Hanford plutonium reprocessing plant (average dose about one rem), and Caldwell, Kelley, and Heath (1980) reported an excess of leukemia in military personnel on maneuvers at a nuclear bomb test. Najarian and Colton (1978) reported a fivefold increase in proportionate mortality due to leukemia and a twofold increase in all cancers at the Portsmouth Naval Shipyard, where nuclear submarines are built. However, their observations were not confirmed in a study requested by a committee of the U.S. House of Representatives (Rinsky, Zumwalde, Waxweiler, et al., 1981). An excess of malignant melanoma has been reported among employees (particularly chemists) at Lawrence Livermore National Laboratory in Berkeley, California (Austin, Reynolds, Snyder, et al., 1981), and there are other reports showing excessive risk at an exposure of about one rad, including studies on ankylosing spondylitics treated with x-rays (Smith & Doll, 1978), on children irradiated for ringworm (Modan, Ron, & Werner, 1977), on persons having diagnostic radiation (Bross, Ball, & Falen, 1979), and on children who received *in utero* radiation (Stewart & Kneale, 1970).

Natural background radiation has traditionally been used as a point of reference for assessing the hazards of other sources of radiation, the assumption being that it represents a safe level. Morgan (1979–1980), however, estimates that 13,000 cancer deaths per year in the United States are attributable to natural background radiation, and several reports indicate that at least radon gas in the natural background poses a significant hazard. Harley (1984, p. 1525) states: "Radon is the gaseous member of the natural radioactive uranium series, and it is formed directly from the decay of radium. Although radon gas itself gives a small radiation dose, it decays into two solid alpha-emitting short-lived daughters; these are inhaled and deposited on the bronchial tree, and they deliver a dose that is carcinogenic."

A recent study (Axelson, Edling, Kling, et al., 1981) on the population of a small Baltic island with a limestone surface soil and a uranium-containing shale underneath showed an excess of lung cancer in the population of that island compared to the expected lung cancer rate in the general population. The excess correlated with the level of exposure to radon daughters, especially in nonwooden houses.

Miners may be exposed to radon emitted by the mine walls. In a study of Swedish iron miners, Radford and Renard (1984) found that among nonsmoking miners there were 18 deaths from lung cancer as compared with 1.8 expected among a comparable population of nonsmoking nonminers. Among miners who were current smokers and recent exsmokers, 32 deaths were observed as compared with the expected 11. Samet, Kutvirt, Waxweiler, and Key (1984) observed a similar excess risk for lung cancer death among Navajo uranium miners. Navajo men are predominantly nonsmokers.

A recent symposium volume (Koval, 1984) reports that the average external radiation we absorb from terrestrial sources has been slightly reduced because of increased indoor living. However, a study of 100 frame houses in Chicago has revealed that forced-air heating spreads the radon uniformly throughout the house from its source in soil gases coming from near and around foundations. The highest 10 percent of these houses were as radon contaminated as those in Grand Junction, Colorado, where builders routinely used uranium mine tailings as backfill. It is concluded that natural background radiation contributes perhaps 1 in 40 of the cancer deaths we now count. On the basis of about 400,000 cancer deaths per year in the United States, about 10,000 may be attributable to natural background radiation (Koval, 1984).

Much of the discussion regarding the issue of maximum permissible exposure has focused on the question of whether or not there is a threshold level below which there is no risk of radiation damage. The data used to support one side or the other in this controversy are derived largely from two sources: animal studies and observations on survivors of the Hiroshima and Nagasaki bombings, the latter carried out by the Atomic Bomb Casualty Commission (ABCC). The reliability of animal studies suffers from the great uncertainty in extrapolating dose–effect data to humans because of species differences in respect to many functions as well as sensitivity to radiation. Moreover, animal studies have been carried out largely on inbred strains, so comparisons between different strains of the same species may not be valid.

The ABCC study is based on an elaborate dosimetry formulation that is based on the distance of survivors from the epicenter of the explosion and takes into account various intervening factors that may have provided shielding. The family registration system virtually guarantees 100-percent mortality follow-up. Nevertheless, the BEIR III Report (1980, pp. 151–157) lists problems that limit the value of the ABCC program, and Marshall (1981a, b) has reported on deliberations concerning the possibility that the estimates of radiation toxicity may have been understated. Schull, Otake, and Neel (1981) also have discussed a reappraisal of genetic effects of the atomic bombs, and one of the authors (Neel, 1981) has editorialized on the need for further studies some three and a half decades after the event. Even so, there have been two additional historical accounts of the ABCC program, one from an American perspective (Councilman, 1980) and the other presenting a Japanese point of view (Ishikawa & Swain, 1981). Figure 4–2, from the Councilman account, is illustrative of the dose–response relationship in respect to the leukemias; and Table 4–8, derived from the Japanese account, provides some data in respect to dose–response relationships for several neoplasms.

The issue of whether or not there is a safe level of radiation exposure has centered on whether dose–response relationships exhibit a linear configuration or take the form of a quadratic curve expressive of an exponential relationship. Figure 4–3 from Morgan (1978) illustrates conditions under which the linear and quadratic forms of dose–response relationships may apply. Morgan (1979–1980, pp. 9–11) points out further that all of the agencies listed in Table 4–7 "have discarded the threshold hypothesis in favor of the linear hypothesis." The BEIR III Report (1980, pp. 141–142) concludes: "This family is the product of a general quadratic ('linear-quadratic') form representing carcinogenesis and an exponential form representing the competing effect of cell-killing often suggested by experimental data in which the observed dose–response has declined at high doses."

The issue of whether or not certain risks are greater at low doses than at high ones has been addressed by Hori and Nakai (1978). They exposed human peripheral blood leukocytes to tritiated water and tritiated thymidine and demonstrated that at higher doses the yields of chromosomal abnormalities increased linearly with each dose. However, the yield at the lower dose range was significantly higher

Figure 4-2 The Combined Incidence of Leukemias at Hiroshima and Nagasaki, Showing a Striking Dose–Response Relationship

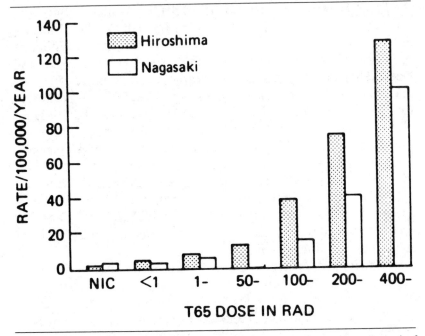

Source: M. Councilman. Hiroshima, Nagasaki, and the RERF. *American Journal of Pathology*, 1980, *98*:843–856. Used with permission.

Table 4-8 Absolute and Relative Risks for Certain Neoplasms in Hiroshima-Nagasaki Survivors (for exposure over 100 rads)

Neoplasm	Overall Absolute Risk	Relative Risk
Leukemia (all types)	2/million/yr./rad	40–50 times normal
Thyroid cancer	4/million/yr./rad	
Lung cancer		Over twice normal
Breast cancer	4/million/yr./rad	6–8 times normal
Stomach cancer	1.2–2.7/million/yr./rad	
Multiple myeloma		4.7 times normal

Source: Data from E. Ishikawa, with D. L. Swain (transl.). *Hiroshima and Nagasaki: The Physical, Medical, and Social Effects of the Atomic Bombings.* New York: Basic Books, 1981.

Figure 4-3 Cancer Induction as a Function of Dose of Ionizing Radiation from 0 to 100 rem

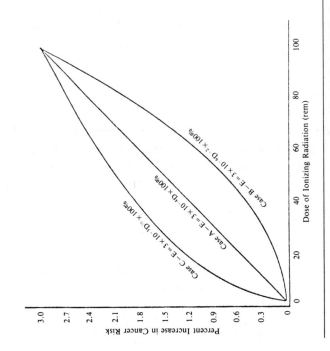

This figure is a plot of equation

$$E = kD^n\%\ \ \ \ \ (1)$$

in which E = cancer risk (percent of persons with cancer) as a result of exposure to a dose D (rem) of ionizing radiation.

Case A, in which n = 1, illustrates the *linear hypothesis* in which one would expect 3×10^{-4} cancers per person.rem.

Case B, in which n = 2, illustrates the old *threshold hypothesis* where the cancer risk becomes negligible or statistically insignificant at low average dose per person. Perhaps it typifies the low leukemia risk of middle-aged persons that are exposed to low LET (linear energy transfer) radiation.

Recent human studies suggest that Case C, or some other curve for which n < 1, applies to leukemia among the young and the old and perhaps to most other forms of cancer irregardless of the age of the person. In such cases the risk per person.rem is greater at low doses than at high doses.

Curves A, B and C are given primarily for illustration, but each curve appears to be applicable in certain cases. Perhaps it is of interest to note that for a dose of 1 rem the cancer risk is 0.03 percent by the linear hypothesis (curve A) and 3×10^{-4} percent (negligible) by the threshold hypothesis (curve B).

Source: K. Z. Morgan. Cancer and Low Level Ionizing Radiation. *Bulletin of the Atomic Scientists,* September 1978, 30–41. Reprinted by permission of THE BULLETIN OF THE ATOMIC SCIENTISTS, a magazine of science and public affairs. Copyright © by the Educational Foundation for Nuclear Science, Chicago, Ill., 60637.

than would be expected by a downward extrapolation from the linear relation. A similar finding in respect to the dose–response relationship was reported by Dobson and Kwan (1976). They provided tritiated water to pregnant mice and then counted the surviving oocytes in their 14-day-old offspring. They also reported a no-threshold effect and a greater-than-expected oocyte killing in the low dose range.

One of the puzzling aspects of the ABCC studies on Japanese survivors is that the incidence of individuals with chromosomal aberrations in cultured lymphocytes is greater than the incidence of malignancy or genetic effects. However, the relationship of these chromosomal aberrations to autoimmune disorders or to lifespan has not been studied adequately. Moreover, the studies with tritiated water just cited are particularly relevant to the issue of whether or not the levels of tritium in the coolant water of nuclear power plants pose a significant risk.

It seems fair to ask whether all of this is an intellectual exercise or is applicable to predicting exposure effects on a human population. The discussion regarding this issue has dealt much less with genetic or lifespan effects than with carcinogenesis and cell killing. The mathematical applications assume a homogeneity of the exposed population that, at best, would hold only for single, inbred animal strains. They would not be valid for comparisons of different inbred strains and certainly not for genetically heterogeneous human populations. Moreover, as Morgan (1978) has noted, human studies have extended over only a small fraction of the lifespan and the applicability of animal data to human populations is highly questionable.

Nor are indirect effects of radiation adequately taken into account. Impairment of DNA repair capacity or of immune function may give rise to infectious disease, autoimmunity, and perhaps a variety of other disorders that have not been considered adequately, perhaps because of a preoccupation with carcinogenesis. As Rotblat (1977) has pointed out, the failure to find a genetic effect among survivors of the Hiroshima–Nagasaki bombings may be due to the fact that a particularly vulnerable segment of the exposed population may have died of infectious disease, particularly pneumonia, as a result of impairment of immune function, leaving a predominantly resistant portion of the population for long-term study.

While "permissible" levels have been reduced considerably over the past several decades as a result of experience gained during that period, there remain doubts as to whether they have been lowered sufficiently to assure safety. It would appear that decisions regarding safety standards have been governed as much by the risks that society is willing to tolerate as by scientific considerations.

CONCLUSION

At the beginning of this chapter, Schubert and Lapp (1958) were quoted as stating that tissues are injured in precisely the same way by excessive radiation, regardless of the source. In pointing out the sources of ionizing radiation and their proportionate contribution to human exposure, it has become apparent that sufficient human-made radiation has been added to natural background radiation, so that, on the average, the two are about equal. Thus, as we prepare to enter the twenty-first century, it can be stated that humans are being exposed to about twice the amount of radiation as 100 years ago, and from an increasing variety of sources.

The effects of ionizing radiation also have been described here. In the main they consist of fetal wastage, congenital and hereditary disorders, carcinogenesis, accelerated aging, reduction or destruction of immune capacity, and possibly impairment of DNA repair mechanisms. All of these effects probably also derive from the same mechanism, the destruction or mutation of genes.

While the probability of radiation damage increases with the level of exposure, there are several additional variables that may determine whether or not an individual develops radiation damage. Included among such variables are the stage of the lifespan at which exposure takes place, differences among species, and even differences among individuals of the same species in a genetically heterogeneous population. It has been pointed out here that, even with a "hit," one individual may have an adequate DNA repair mechanism or a level of immune capacity to compensate for the radiation lesion, while another may be deficient in such mechanisms and develop a radiation-related disorder. It also has been pointed out that in determining effects on population exposures, such as those connected with the Hiroshima–Nagasaki bombings, the most susceptible segment of the population may succumb early because of damage to the immune system and the consequent development of infectious disease, particularly pneumonia. This would leave for long-term study the "fittest" of the population and therefore produce an underestimation of the overall frequency of a lesion such as cancer or genetic defect.

Mathematical constructs have been used extensively in an attempt to establish safe levels of radiation exposure, that is, a maximum permissible dose. While it may appear that major regulatory bodies have abandoned the threshold concept, we still retain a policy of applying maximum permissible exposures that are about 10 times higher for radiation workers than for the general population. These mathematical constructs have been used, for the most part, to predict the approximate number of cancer cases from a given exposure. It now is well established that cancer develops through a series of stages that include initiation and promotion and that different environmental agents may act in consort. Thus, in order to predict the frequency of carcinogenesis from a given exposure, it also would be necessary to know the frequency of concomitant exposure to agents other than ionizing radiation—such as cigarette consumption, dietary factors, and chemical pollutants—that may act as co-carcinogens (see Chapter 1).

When one considers all of the variables necessary for an accurate prediction of damage likely to accrue from a given radiation exposure, it becomes evident that no study to date has included all possible factors and indeed it may not even be possible to design a study that would accomplish this purpose. If one accepts the "no threshold" hypothesis and the estimate of 13,000 cancer cases per year from natural background radiation, then average radiation exposure at present levels may account for at least 26,000 cases per year. In the final analysis, however, decisions regarding permissible levels have not been made on the basis of scientific considerations alone, but rather on an assessment of a so-called cost–benefit (or risk–benefit) ratio, that is, on the basis of how many radiation-related deaths society is willing to tolerate for the benefits that may accrue from the use of ionizing radiation.

Schneider and Morton (1981) present as the central thesis of their book that, while the solution to problems such as those posed by nuclear energy may appear purely technical, they cannot be dealt with only on the basis of scientific information and cost–benefit analysis. Their true solution requires an understanding of sociocultural beliefs and humanistic values. Few scientists would argue that exposure to low-level irradiation is completely safe or that such exposure can be made completely safe. Scientists do, however, have differing views as to the extent of risk as well as the cost–benefit ratio. An important consideration in respect to the latter is how properly to insert humanistic values into the question. What is the dollar value of a human life, how many lives are to be sacrificed on the altar of nuclear power, and whose lives are they to be?

REFERENCES

Anderson, R. K., and Lefkovits, I. (1979). In vitro evaluation of radiation-induced augmentation of the immune response. *Am. J. Pathol. 97*:456–472.

Austin, D. F., Reynolds, P. J., Snyder, M. A., Biggs, M. W., and Stubbs, H. A. (1981). Malignant melanoma among employees of Lawrence Livermore National Laboratory. *Lancet 2*:712–717.

Axelson, O., Edling, C., Kling, H., Anderson, L., and Ringner, A. (1981). Lung cancer and radon in dwellings. *Lancet 2*:995–996.

Baverstock, K. F., Papworth, D., and Vennart, J. (1981). Risk of radiation at low dose rates. *Lancet 1*:430–433.

BEIR III Report (Committee on the Biological Effects of Ionizing Radiations) (1980). *The Effects on Populations of Exposure to Low Levels of Ionizing Radiation.* Washington, D.C.: National Academy Press.

Benditt, E. P., and Benditt, J. M. (1973). Evidence for a monoclonal origin of human atherosclerotic plaques. *Proc. Nat. Acad. Sci. USA 70*:1753–1756.

Bizzozero, O. J. Jr., Johnson, K. G., and Ciocco, A. (1966). Radiation related leukemia in Hiroshima and Nagasaki, 1946–1964. 1. Distribution, incidence and appearance time. *New Eng. J. Med. 274*:1095–1101.

Blumenthal, H. T. (1983). The aging-disease connection in retrospect and prospect. In H. T. Blumenthal (ed.), *Handbook of Diseases of Aging.* New York: Van Nostrand Reinhold.

Bross, I. D. J., Ball, M., and Falen, S. (1979). A dosage response curve for the one rad range: Adult risks from diagnostic radiation. *Am. J. Publ. Health 69*:130–136.

Burnet, F. M. (1983). Age-associated heredo-degenerative conditions of the nervous system. In H. T. Blumenthal (ed.), *Handbook of Aging.* New York: Van Nostrand Reinhold.

Caldwell, L. G., Kelley, D. B., and Heath, C. W. Jr. (1980). Leukemia among participants in military maneuvers at a nuclear bomb test: A preliminary report. *JAMA 244*:1575–1578.

Casarett, G. L. (1981). Out of sites. *The Sciences 21* (May–June):18–30.

Councilman, M. (1980). Hiroshima, Nagasaki, and the RERF. *Am. J. Pathol. 98*: 843–856.

Court Brown, W. J., and Doll, R. (1965). Mortality from cancer and other causes after radiotherapy for ankylosing spondylitis. *Brit. Med. J.* 2:1327–1332.

Curtis, H. J. (1966). *Biological Mechanisms of Aging.* Springfield, Ill.: Charles C Thomas.

Curtis, H. J., and Gebhard, K. L. (1958). Comparison of life-shortening effects of toxic and radiation stresses. *Radiation Res* 9:104.

Dobson, R. L., and Cooper, M. E. (1974). Tritium toxicity: Effect of low level ³HOH exposure on developing female germ cells in the mouse. *Radiation Res.* 58:91–100.

Dobson, R. L., and Kwan, T. C. (1976). The RBE of tritium radiation measured in mouse oocytes: Increase at low exposure levels. *Radiation Res.* 66:615–625.

Emerson, C. H., and Braverman, L. E. (1980). Thyroid irradiation — one view. *New Eng. J. Med. 303*:217–219.

Failla, B. (1958). The aging process and carcinogenesis. *Ann. N.Y. Acad. Sci.* 71:1124–1135.

Gabbay, K. H. (1980). The insulinopathies. *New Eng. J. Med. 302*:165–167.

Harley, N. H. (1984). Editorial: Radon and lung cancer in mines and homes. *New Eng. J. Med. 310*:1525–1526.

Harting, F. H., and Hesse, W. (1879). Der Lungskrebs: die Bergkrankheit in den Schneeberger Gruben. *Viertelj. für Gerichtl. Med. u. offen Sanitats.* 30:296–308; 31:102–132; 313–337.

Hori, T. A., and Nakai, S. (1978). Unusual dose-response of chromosome aberrations induced in human lymphocytes by very low dose exposures to tritium. *Mutation Res.* 50:101–110.

Ishikawa, E., with Swain, D. L. (transl.) (1981). *Hiroshima and Nagasaki: The Physical, Medical and Social Effects of the Atomic Bombings.* By the Committee for the Compilation of Materials on Damage Caused by the Atomic Bombs in Hiroshima and Nagasaki. New York: Basic Books.

Jacobs, P. A., Court Brown, W. M., and Doll, R. (1961). Distribution of human chromosome counts in relation to age. *Nature 191*:1178–1180.

Janigan, D. T., and Druet, R. L. (1968). Experimental murine amyloidosis in x-irradiated recipients of spleen homogenates or serum from sensitized donors. *Am. J. Pathol.* 52:381–390.

Kellum, M. J., Sutherland, D. E. R., Eckert, E., Peterson, D. A., and Good, R. A. (1965). Wasting disease, Coombs-positivity, and amyloidosis in rabbits subjected to central lymphoid tissue extirpation and irradiation. *Int. Arch. Allergy* 27:6–26.

Koval, T. M. (1984). *Environmental Radioactivity.* Proceedings of the Nineteenth Annual Meeting of the National Council on Radiation Protection and Measurements, Bethesda Maryland, April 6–7, 1983.

Lesher, S., Grahn, D., and Sallese, A. (1957). Amyloidosis in mice exposed to daily gamma irradiation. *J. Natl. Cancer Inst.* 19:1119–1127.

Lindop, P. (1981). Quoted by Weinberg, A. M., in review of *The Fast Breeder Reactor: Need? Cost?* (London: Macmillan Press, 1980), *Nature 289*:519.

Mancuso, T. F., Stewart, A. M., and Kneale, G. W. (1977). Radiation exposure of Hanford workers dying from cancer and other causes. *Health Physics 33*:369–385.

Marshall, E. (1981a). News and comment: New A-bomb studies alter radiation estimates. *Science 212*:900–903.

Marshall, E. (1981b). New A-bomb data shown to radiation experts. *Science 212*:1364–1365.

Matanoski, G. M., Seltser, R., Sartwell, P. E., Diamond, E. L., and Elliott E. A. (1975a). The current mortality rates of radiologists and other physician specialists. Deaths from all causes and from cancer. *Am. J. Epidemiol. 101*:188–198.

Matanoski, G. M., Seltser, R., Sartwell, P. E., Diamond, E. L., and Elliott, E. A. (1975b). The current mortality rates of radiologists and other physician specialists. Specific causes of death. *Am. J. Epidemiol. 101*:199–210.

Modan, B., Ron, E., and Werner, A. (1977). Thyroid cancer following scalp irradiation. *Radiol. 123*:741–744.

Morgan, K. Z. (1978). Cancer and low level ionizing radiation. *Bull. Atomic Sci.* September:30–41.

Morgan, K. Z. (1979–1980). Appreciation of risks of low level radiation vs. nuclear energy. Transcript of paper presented at panel of Natl. Acad. Sci. Sept. 27 and before State-of-the-Art-in-Biology Sympos., Athens, Georgia, Jan. 11, 1980.

Musacchia, X. J., and Blumenthal, H. T. (unpublished). Acceleration of the development of senile amyloidosis in the golden hamster by x-irradiation.

Najarian, T., and Colton, T. (1978). Mortality from leukemia and cancer in shipyard nuclear workers. *Lancet 1*:1018–1020.

Neel, J. V. (1981). Editorial: Genetic effects of atomic bombs. *Science 213*:1205.

Peters, M., Mackay, I. R., and Buckley, J. D. (1980). Occurrence of tumors and effects on longevity after limited x-irradiation in man. *Am. J. Pathol. 101*:647–656.

Radford, E. P., and Renard, K. G. St.C. (1984). Lung cancer in Swedish iron miners exposed to low doses of radon daughters. *New Eng. J. Med. 310*: 1485–1494.

Rinsky, R. A., Zumwalde, R. D., Waxweiler, R. J., Murray, W. E. Jr., Bierbaum, P. J., Landrigan, P. J., Terpilak, M., and Cox, C. (1981). Cancer mortality at a naval nuclear shipyard. *Lancet 1*:231–235.

Rotblat, J. (1977). The puzzle of absent effects. *New Scientist 75*:475–476.

Rotwein, P., Chyn, R., Chirgwin, J., Cordell, B., Goodman, H. M., and Permutt, M. A. (1981). Polymorphism in the 5′-flanking region of the human insulin gene and its possible relation to type 2 diabetes. *Science 213*:1117–1120.

Samet, J. M., Kutvirt, D. M., Waxweiler, R. J., and Key, C. R. (1984). Uranium mining and lung cancer in Navajo men. *New Eng. J. Med. 310*:1481–1484.

Schneider, S. H., and Morton, L. (1981). *The Primordial Bond: Exploring Connections between Man and Nature through the Humanities and Science.* New York: Plenum.

Schubert, J., and Lapp, R. E. (1958). *Radiation. What It Is and How It Affects You.* New York: Viking Press.

Schull, W. J., Otake, M., and Neel, J. V. (1981). Genetic effects of the atomic bomb: A reappraisal. *Science 213*:1220–1227.

Seltser, R., and Sartwell, P. E. (1965). The influence of occupational exposure to radiation on the mortality of American radiologists and other medical specialists. *Am. J. Epidemiol. 81*:2–22.

Smith, P. G., and Doll, R. (1978). Age and time-dependent changes in the rates of radiation-induced cancers in patients with ankylosing spondylitis following a single course of x-ray treatment. *Internat. Atomic Agency Report* (Vienna) SM-224/711.

Stewart, A., and Kneale, G. W. (1970). Radiation dose effects in relation to obstetric x-rays and childhood cancers. *Lancet 1*:1185–1188.

Szilard, L. (1959). On the nature of the aging process. *Proc. Natl. Acad. Sci. USA 45*:30–42.

Van Cleave, C. D. (1968). *Late Somatic Effects of Ionizing Irradiation.* Springfield, Va.: Div. Technical Information, U.S. Atomic Energy Comm. Natl. Bureau of Standards, U.S. Dept. Commerce.

Warren, S. (1956). Longevity and causes of death from irradiation in physicians. *JAMA 162*:464–468.

Weksler, M. E. (1981). The senescence of the immune system. *Hosp. Practice 16*:53–64.

Chapter 5

Air Pollution

Daniel S. Blumenthal
Milford Greene

Air pollution has always been with us. Naturally occurring phenomena such as volcanic eruptions, tree and grass pollination, and swamp gas have always tainted the air. The environment, however, is armed with natural mechanisms for dealing with these acts of nature.

Historically, concern for the effects of air pollution on health dates back to at least the thirteenth century. In England, between 1285 and 1310, several government commissions were established to investigate sources of air pollution and the fouling of air that accompanied a shift from wood to coal as the principal fuel in lime kilns.

Air pollution increased as a concern during the Industrial Revolution, a term usually applied to the sudden and remarkable series of changes that occurred in industry in England between 1760 and 1790. A parallel period of industrialization occurred in the United States in the 30-year period beginning in 1808, when a series of political events led to the development of manufacturing by the factory system, in addition to the agriculture and commerce that existed already. The first smoke-control laws in this country were established in Cincinnati and Chicago in 1881, and 23 of the 28 largest cities had passed laws by 1912 (Council on Environmental Quality, 1970).

The adverse effects of air-borne pollutants are many. They include damage to:

1. *Human health*. Air pollution may cause both acute effects, as in major air pollution episodes, as well as chronic effects secondary to low levels of pollutants. Air pollution has been implicated in the course of such diseases as asthma, bronchitis, cancer, cardiovascular disease, and emphysema. Increased mortality rates have been attributed to air pollution in several smog episodes. Air pollution also is implicated as a cause of adverse health effects on animals.
2. *Vegetation and agricultural output*. Various pollutants damage flowers and food plants, and luxuriant forests have been completely destroyed by fumes from copper smelters and other industrial sources.
3. *Property*. Materials such as paint on cars and houses are blackened or corroded by hydrogen sulfide; rubber is cracked by ozone; some metals are corroded by sulfur dioxide.
4. *Aesthetics*. Many pollutants are malodorous and affect visibility. Particulate matter in the atmosphere and photochemical smog have impaired visibility so badly at airports that they have been considered to be a serious aircraft hazard.
5. *The economy*. Air pollution is a cause of increased absenteeism, morbidity, hospitalization, mortality, decreased working efficiency, and crop and property destruction.
6. *Weather*. Increased particulate concentrations in the atmosphere have resulted in the seeding of clouds and increased rainfall.

WEATHER, CLIMATE, AND AIR POLLUTION

An understanding of some of the fundamentals of meteorology — in particular, the movements of air masses and the factors that influence these movements — is essential to an appreciation of the mechanisms by which air pollutants accumulate, are dispersed, and come into contact with humans (Corman, 1978).

The atmosphere surrounding the earth is divided conventionally into four layers. Starting with the layer closest to the earth's surface, these are the troposphere, the stratosphere, the mesosphere, and the thermosphere. The majority of meteorological events affecting air pollution takes place in the inner layer, or troposphere. Over 90 percent of the atmosphere's total air mass is concentrated in this 12-mile-thick layer. The size of the troposphere, relative to the earth, is the size of the skin of an apple relative to the apple itself. It is somewhat thinner at the poles of the earth and thicker at the equator.

Movement of air within the troposphere and other layers is related directly to how energy from the sun warms the earth's atmosphere. This is done by three mechanisms: radiation, conduction, and convection. Little of the sun's radiant energy is absorbed by the air directly; rather, this energy is absorbed by the earth and then radiated. Much of the reradiated energy is absorbed by the atmosphere, largely because of its water vapor content.

Conduction—the mechanical transfer of heat energy from one molecule to another—plays a larger role in warming the atmosphere. Heat energy is conducted from the warmed surface of the earth to the adjacent air layer and thence to air layers at higher altitudes.

Convection consists of the transfer of heat by the movement of air masses. Air warmed at the earth's surface expands, becomes lighter, and rises; the cooler air above it then sinks to take its place. Convection, in combination with the rotation of the earth on its axis, is responsible for the patterns of winds in the troposphere. By regularly presenting the sun with a different portion of the earth's surface, the earth's rotation is responsible for the establishment of the prevailing winds (easterlies, westerlies, trades).

The rate at which pollutants in the troposphere are dispersed is governed largely by the air's horizontal movement (wind) and its vertical movement (convection). As air rises and the atmospheric pressure drops, the air expands and becomes cooler. The rate at which it cools is known as the *adiabatic lapse rate*. If this rate is high, warm air rises quickly; under such "unstable" conditions, pollutants are dispersed rapidly. Conversely, under "stable" conditions in which the adiabatic lapse rate is low, pollutants may accumulate.

The vertical distance through which warm air rises while undergoing adiabatic cooling, before it meets air of equal temperature, is the *mixing depth*. This represents the upper limit of pollution dispersion. At times when the earth and its adjacent air layer are relatively cool—as in winter, or at night—the mixing depth is diminished and pollutants may be poorly dispersed.

An *inversion* represents a particularly stable situation in which the surface air is cooler than the layer of air above it and thus cannot rise. Pollutants in this circumstance are effectively trapped close to the surface of the earth. Two types of inversion are of particular importance. A *subsidence inversion* occurs when a layer of air in a high-pressure air mass sinks, is compressed (and thus heated), and traps the cooler air beneath it. Subsidence inversions occur commonly on the west coast of the United States. The second important type of inversion, the *radiation inversion*, occurs frequently on cool nights. As the ground cools (by radiating its heat), the air next to it also cools. Generally, the inversion is broken up as the sun warms the earth in the morning.

Season and topography affect the formation of inversions. Inversions are most persistent during the fall and winter; they are most frequent and most persistent in valleys. Fog often forms in the cool surface air of inversions and can worsen coexisting pollution by, for instance, converting gaseous SO_2 to sulfuric acid mist.

Some related special meteorological effects occurring in urban areas also deserve mention. The numerous vertical concrete surfaces of large city buildings tend to retain heat and create a rising column of warm air over the city center (the heat island effect). This air then cools and settles at the city's periphery. Suspended particulates in the air are thus transported in such a way that they form a dome over the city (dust dome or haze hood). This dome reflects the sun's heat and creates a system that tends to trap pollution in the urban atmosphere (Corman, 1978).

These various meteorological phenomena, on several occasions during the past 50 years, have combined with periods of high pollution to create a number of major acute air pollution episodes. The study of these episodes has contributed considerably to current knowledge of air pollution and its effects on human health.

ACUTE AIR POLLUTION EPISODES

While concern with air pollution on an aesthetic basis dates back several centuries, the first widespread appreciation that this environmental problem can have life-threatening effects stemmed from several acute episodes in the mid twentieth century. Most of the adverse health consequences of these episodes have been attributed to high concentrations of sulfur dioxide and particulates.

The first of these tragedies to arouse worldwide concern occurred in Belgium, in the Meuse River Valley, where a heavily industrialized area extends for some 15 miles. The terrain has a valley topography, typically lending itself to thermal inversions. Thus, it is no surprise that the Meuse Valley suffered exceedingly when all of Belgium was blanketed by a thick, cold fog in the first week of December, 1930. Trapped by the inversion, the pollutants gathered day after day and stagnated. Within a few days, thousands fell ill; 63 persons died from the poisoned air. The dead were mostly the elderly and those already very ill from diseases of the heart or lungs. Those who merely sickened complained quickly of coughing and shortness of breath (Firket, 1931).

Donora, Pennsylvania was the victim of a similar situation. The town, crammed with industry, is located in the Monongahela River Valley. In October 1948, during an inversion that covered a wide area of the northeastern United States, Donora had its tragedy. Among a population of only 14,000, close to 6000 fell ill. Instead of the expected two deaths for the period, the fog and pollutant-filled inversion produced 20. Again, the elderly were hit harder and more frequently; again, preexisting heart or lung disease was a frequent concomitant; and again, most people coughed—although they also suffered sore throats, dyspnea, headaches, burning and tearing eyes, running noses, nausea, and vomiting (Schrenk, Heimann, Clayton, et al., 1949).

London has had several acute episodes. The worst of these occurred in December 1952 (Logan, 1953). For centuries, Londoners had heated their homes with soft coal in open fireplaces. The resultant smoke combined with the city's natural fog to create the original "smog." In the 1952 episode, this smog combined with industrial emissions during a five-day inversion; the resulting acute pollution episode took the lives of an estimated 4000 people. The weekly morbidity rate more than doubled, as well. The normal number of weekly applications for emergency bed service in December in London was about 1000, but during the 1952 episode this number rose to more than 2500. The hospital bed demand did not subside to normal for two to three weeks afterward. As in the other reported episodes, both illness and death struck more often at the elderly and at those with preexisting heart and lung conditions.

Six previous London episodes had been recorded, dating as far back as 1873, with deaths attributed to them totaling over 2500. It is possible, furthermore, that only the precautions brought about by the earlier calamities kept mortality figures down in a similar inversion in December 1962. At that time the deaths of a "mere" 750 people were attributed to polluted air (Scott, 1963).

In New York City, epidemiologic analyses of mortality rates and meteorologic patterns have revealed a number of acute air pollution events, including episodes in 1953, 1962, 1963, and 1966. These episodes were characterized by periods of high pollution levels, temperature inversions, and low winds. Because of the absence of accompanying fog, however, the episodes were not necessarily apparent at the time of their occurrence. In 1953, 200 excess deaths were attributed to an air pollution episode (Greenburg, Jacobs, Drolette, et al., 1963); in 1963, there were 405 excess deaths (McCarroll & Bradley, 1966); and in 1966, 168 excess deaths. The fatalities in the 1966 episode were probably much lower than they might have been because the inversion occurred during a Thanksgiving weekend, when many pollution-producing activities were not carried on, and because certain air pollution restrictions were imposed by the city.

DEFENSE OF THE RESPIRATORY SYSTEM AGAINST AIR-BORNE POLLUTANTS

Claude Bernard, a nineteenth-century physiologist, coined the phrase "inner environment" in 1877 and became one of the first known environmentalists. Bernard was amazed by how well the inner environment of the human body is maintained, given the extremes of the outer environment.

The three major surfaces of the human body with which the outer environment comes into direct contact are the skin, the gastrointestinal tract, and the respiratory tract. Although the irritant materials of air pollution affect the skin and the gastrointestinal system, the major effect on health is the result of these materials acting on the respiratory tract. The entire surface area of the respiratory tract ranges between 80 and 100 square meters, approximately the size of a tennis court.

One of the major functions of the respiratory system is accomplished through the phenomenon of cell respiration, a series of exergonic cellular processes in which organic substances are oxidized and chemical energy is released. Lavoisier, in 1780, demonstrated that animals use oxygen from the air and produce carbon dioxide. In order to carry out this process, an individual inspires some 10,000 to 20,000 liters of air per day, each liter of which may contain several million suspended particles.

Inspired air follows a pathway through the nasal and oral passages, the trachea, bronchi, and bronchioles and eventually into the pulmonary alveoli where oxygen is extracted and taken up by the red blood cells. The highly compartmentalized surface area of the lungs is composed of some 300 million tiny alveoli. Air-borne pollutants against which the body must defend itself may be either particulate or gaseous.

Particulate Pollutants

The cleansing of the lungs of air-borne particles is accomplished by two basic defense mechanisms: *deposition* and *clearance.*

Deposition is the process by which inhaled air-borne particles are caught on cell surfaces in the proximal portions of the respiratory tract and fail to exit with expired air. Essentially all particulate matter deposits upon touching a respiratory surface; the initial point of contact is the point of deposition.

Deposition is affected by three distinct physical phenomena that operate on suspended inspired particulates and influence their movement toward the surface of the respiratory tract. These are *inertia, sedimentation,* and *Brownian diffusion.* Inertia denotes the resistance of an inspired particle to changes in speed and direction of air flow. The respiratory tract has repeated branches and sudden changes in direction of air flow. Inertial forces tend to propel large particles in the same direction and at the same speed as when inspired, causing the particles to contact the walls of the respiratory tract. Sedimentation results from the pull of gravity on suspended particles. The sedimentation velocity is determined by the difference between gravitational forces and viscous resistive forces. The third force, Brownian diffusion, is a random motion caused by molecular collisions. This tends to cause very small particles to move across air streams and increases the probability that they will deposit.

How well a particle deposits is dependent upon three factors:

1. The anatomy of the respiratory tract
2. The effective aerodynamic diameters of the inspired particles
3. The pattern of breathing

Anatomical factors include airway diameter, the number and kinds of angles an inspired particle encounters, and the distance an inspired particle must travel to the alveolar walls. The velocity of the air stream is also important and can vary with a switch from nose to mouth breathing and with any change in the volume of the lung as a result of aging and/or disease.

The effective aerodynamic diameter of an inspired particle is a function of its size, shape, and density. Inertia and sedimentation primarily influence the rate at which large particles deposit; Brownian diffusion acts chiefly on the smallest particles.

Breathing patterns will determine the air flow velocity and, to an extent, the number of inspired particles. The volume and frequency of inspiration will affect the length of time a particle is in the respiratory tract and hence the probability of deposition as a result of gravitational and diffusional forces.

The second protective mechanism for particulates, clearance, is the dynamic process that physically expels an inspired particle once it is deposited. If however, a particle is highly soluble, it will dissolve and become absorbed into the blood stream. Thereafter, it may be metabolized and excreted.

Clearance takes place at three distinct levels within the respiratory tract:

1. The upper respiratory tract (nasopharynx)
2. The tracheobronchial tree
3. The pulmonary alveoli

In the nasopharynx, the deposition of inspired particles occurs on fine hairs and in the narrow and tortuous passages of the nose. Clearance is accomplished by nose blowing, sneezing, coughing, mucociliary action, and swallowing.

Particles that impact the ciliated regions of the nasopharynx and are not very soluble deposit on a mucous blanket that covers the airways and moves particles toward the pharynx. There they mix with saliva and are swallowed. The mucous blanket is critically important to clearance in this region of the respiratory tract, and intrinsic and extrinsic factors that affect ciliary action can modify the rate at which an irritant is cleared.

In the tracheobronchial tree, inspired particles are removed from the air stream by sedimentation and diffusion. Once a particle is deposited, it is cleared by coughing or mucociliary action or is absorbed by bronchial blood flow.

Air-borne particles that become deposited in the lower nonciliated alveolar zone of the respiratory tract may be phagocytized or moved in the direction of the ciliated epithelium by alveolar macrophages. These cells act to decrease the probability of particle penetration of the alveolar wall. They also may play a role in the development of emphysema and other pulmonary diseases, however. When injured or dying, they leak proteolytic enzymes; this process has been implicated in the pathogenesis of emphysema (Bates, 1972). In addition, they tend to concentrate irritants and toxins into "hot spots," magnifying their pathogenic effects.

Particles not otherwise cleared may be carried by transepithelial transport to the lymph and blood stream. Although removed from the respiratory tree, these particles may do damage elsewhere in the body.

Gaseous Pollutants

Neuroreceptors located throughout the respiratory tree provide a first line of defense against inspired toxic gases. Stimulation of different receptors results in coughing, sneezing, laryngospasm, bronchoconstriction, or tachypnea. The rate of absorption of inspired gases is a function of their solubility and chemical reactivity as well as the rate and depth of respiration. More soluble gases, such as SO_2, are largely absorbed in the upper airways, where they may be buffered, detoxified, diffused into the circulation, or exert a local toxic effect. Less soluble gases, such as NO_2 and O_3, pass more deeply into the respiratory tract. Despite their relatively low solubility, the large alveolar surface area of the human lung results in fairly efficient absorption. Nonirritant gases such as CO bypass the defense mechanisms of the upper airway and are well absorbed.

AIR POLLUTANTS AND THEIR SOURCES

The 1970 amendments to the Clean Air Act required the U.S. Environmental Protection Agency (EPA) to establish National Ambient Air Quality Standards (NAAQS) for certain pollutants. These "criteria" pollutants, for which standards have been established, are: photochemical oxidants (or ozone, O_3); carbon monoxide (CO); sulfur dioxide (SO_2); total suspended particulates (TSP); nitrogen dioxide (NO_2); hydrocarbons (HC); and lead (Pb). For each of these, as shown in Table 5-1, the EPA has set "primary standards" designed to protect human health with a reasonable margin of safety, as well as "secondary standards," designed to protect against effects on human welfare such as crop losses or metal corrosion. In addition, several other air pollutants are thought to represent hazards to human health. These include heavy metals, asbestos, radionuclides, and specific organic chemicals.

Although humans are usually exposed to multiple pollutants simultaneously and these substances may act synergistically, it is useful to consider briefly the sources and actions of individual pollutants.

Ozone (O_3).   This is a poisonous form of pure oxygen and the principal component of modern smog. Until recently, EPA called this type of pollution "photochemical oxidants." The name was changed because ozone was the only oxidant actually measured and by far the most plentiful.

Ozone and other oxidants—including peroxyacetal nitrates (PAN), formaldehyde, and peroxides—are not emitted into the air directly. They are formed by chemical reactions in the air from two other pollutants, hydrocarbons and nitrogen oxides. Energy from sunlight is needed for these chemical reactions (hence the term photochemical smog), resulting in daily variations in ozone levels, increasing during the day and decreasing at night.

Ozone is a respiratory irritant; exposure produces histologic changes in the lung, including fibrosis and thickening of the alveolar wall (Freeman, Juhos, Furiosi, et al., 1974). Two-hour exposures in the range of 500 to 1480 $\mu g/m^3$ produce impaired pulmonary function in lightly exercising human subjects (Hackney, Linn, Karuza, et al., 1977). Intense exposure may result in pulmonary edema.

Carbon Monoxide.   This is a colorless, odorless, poisonous gas formed when carbon-containing fuel is not burned completely.

Table 5-1 National Ambient Air Quality Standards

Pollutant	Averaging Time	Primary Standard Levels	Secondary Standard Levels
Particulate matter	Annual (geometric mean)	75 $\mu g/m^3$	60 $\mu g/m^3$
	24 hrs[b]	260 $\mu g/m^3$	150 $\mu g/m^3$
Sulfur oxides	Annual (arithmetic mean)	80 $\mu g/m^3$ (0.03 ppm)	— —
	24 hrs[b]	365 $\mu g/m^3$ (0.14 ppm)	— —
	3 hrs[b]	— —	1300 $\mu g/m^3$ (0.5 ppm)
Carbon monoxide	8 hrs[b]	10 mg/m^3 (9 ppm)	10 mg/m^3 (9 ppm)
	1 hr[b]	40 mg/m^3 * (35 ppm)	40 mg/m^3 * (35 ppm)
Nitrogen dioxide	Annual (arithmetic mean)	100 $\mu g/m^3$ (0.05 ppm)	100 $\mu g/m^3$ (0.05 ppm)
Ozone	1 hr[b]	240 $\mu g/m^3$ (0.12 ppm)	240 $\mu g/m^3$ (0.12 ppm)
Hydrocarbons (nonmethane)[a]	3 hrs (6 to 9 A.M.)	160 $\mu g/m^3$ (0.24 ppm)	160 $\mu g/m^3$ (0.24 ppm)
Lead	3 mos	1.5 $\mu g/m^3$	1.5 $\mu g/m^3$

* EPA has proposed a reduction of the standard to 25 ppm (29 mg/m^3).

[a] A nonhealth-related standard used as a guide for ozone control.

[b] Not to be exceeded more than once a year.

Source: Council on Environmental Quality. *Environmental Quality 1981.* Washington, D.C.: U.S. Government Printing Office, 1982.

It is by far the most plentiful air pollutant. EPA estimates that more than 85 million metric tons of CO are emitted into the air each year in the United States. Fortunately, this toxic gas does not persist in the atmosphere. It is converted by natural processes to carbon dioxide, in ways not yet understood, quickly enough to prevent widespread accumulation. It can reach dangerous levels in local areas, however. More than 75 percent of the CO emitted comes from road vehicles (see Table 5-2).

Carbon monoxide is an asphyxiant that binds with hemoglobin to form carboxyhemoglobin, displacing oxygen from the red blood cells. At relatively low exposure levels (79 to 97 mg/m^3 for one hour), CO can decrease exercise tolerance in patients with coronary artery disease (Aronow & Isbell, 1973). In sufficient quantity, it is rapidly fatal.

Sulfur Dioxide and Total Suspended Particulates.   Sulfur dioxide and suspended particulates generally are considered together as the sulfur dioxide/particulate complex. This is because the two pollutants usually are found together in urban settings and because SO_2 itself is transformed in the atmosphere into a particulate sulfate aerosol. Other particulates include dust, soot, smoke, and a number of chemicals of varying toxicity, including oxides of carbon, iron, aluminum, silicon, and phosphorus.

Combustion of fossil fuels is the chief source of the sulfur dioxide/particulate complex. Its constituents have both irritant and toxic effects on the airways; human exposure results in bronchoconstriction (Weir & Bromberg, 1972) and exacerbation of preexisting pulmonary disease. Increased levels of the complex during acute air pollution episodes have been associated with increased mortality and exacerbation of cardiac as well as pulmonary disease.

Nitrogen Dioxide (NO$_2$).   This is an oxidation product of nitric oxide (NO), which is produced from atmospheric nitrogen and oxygen under conditions of high-temperature combustion as in engines and boilers. It has irritant and toxic effects on respiratory epithelium but is less acutely toxic than ozone. Acute exposure causes bronchoconstriction in individuals with preexisting lung disease (Orehek, Massari, Garrard, et al., 1976); chronic exposure causes histopathologic changes in animal models (Freeman, Stephes, Crane, & Furiosi, 1968) and may cause increased susceptibility to respiratory infections (Melia, Florey, Altman, & Swan, 1977).

Table 5-2 National Air Pollutant Emissions, by Pollutant and Source, 1980 (million metric tons per year)

Source	Particulates	Sulfur Oxides	Nitrogen Oxides	Hydro-carbons	Carbon Monoxide
TRANSPORTATION	1.4	0.9	9.1	7.8	69.1
Highway vehicles	1.1	0.4	6.6	6.4	61.9
Aircraft	0.1	0.0	0.1	0.2	1.0
Railroads	0.1	0.1	0.7	0.2	0.3
Vessels	0.0	0.3	0.2	0.5	1.5
Other off-highway vehicles	0.1	0.1	1.5	0.5	4.4
STATIONARY SOURCE FUEL					
COMBUSTION	1.4	19.0	10.6	0.2	2.1
Electric utilities	0.8	15.9	6.7	0.0	0.3
Industrial	0.3	2.3	3.3	0.1	0.6
Commercial-institutional	0.1	0.6	0.3	0.0	0.1
Residential	0.2	0.2	0.3	0.1	1.1
INDUSTRIAL PROCESSES	3.7	3.8	0.7	10.8	5.8
SOLID WASTE DISPOSAL	0.4	0.0	0.1	0.6	2.2
Incineration	0.2	0.0	0.0	0.3	1.2
Open burning	0.2	0.0	0.1	0.3	1.0
MISCELLANEOUS	0.9	0.0	0.2	2.4	6.2
Forest fires	0.8	0.0	0.2	0.7	5.5
Other burning	0.1	0.0	0.0	0.1	0.7
Miscellaneous organic solvents	0.0	0.0	0.0	1.6	0.0
TOTAL	7.8	23.7	20.7	21.8	85.4

Source: Council on Environmental Quality. *Environmental Quality 1981.* Washington, D.C.: U.S. Government Printing Office, 1982.

Lead.   Lead is a toxic heavy metal that primarily affects the hematopoetic, renal, and central nervous systems. It accumulates in the body and is stored in bone. Exposure to air-borne lead occurs directly by inhalation or indirectly by ingestion of lead-contaminated food, water, or nonfood materials such as soil and dust.

There are myriad sources of lead exposure other than contaminated air. Concentrated sources include chips of lead-base paint that may be ingested by preschool children living in dilapidated housing; old storage batteries in battery-recycling plants; and moonshine whiskey distilled in apparati constructed from old automobile radiators. Other sources include inks, pesticides, water distribution systems, and some pottery glazes. For the general U.S. population, however, air-borne lead is probably the leading source of exposure.

Lead is emitted primarily by automobiles and other vehicles burning leaded gasoline; in addition, certain industries — for instance, lead and copper smelters (Landrigan, Baker, Feldman, et al., 1976) and battery plants — produce lead emissions. In 1975, gasoline combustion accounted for 90 percent of air-borne lead. EPA regulation of lead in gasoline and controls on the automotive industry have reduced this to slightly over 60 percent presently. As a result of this reduction in air-borne lead, the mean blood lead level of the U.S. population has been reduced 36.7 percent from 15.8 μg/dl in 1976 to 10.0 μg/dl in 1980 (*Morbidity and Mortality Weekly Report*, 1982).

Hydrocarbons.   Hydrocarbons are compounds of varying complexity consisting of two elements, hydrogen and carbon. The simplest hydrocarbon, methane (CH_4), is not included in atmospheric hydrocarbon measurements.

Most of the estimated 28 million metric tons of hydrocarbons emitted each year in the United States comes from gasoline that is incompletely burned in automobile engines or evaporates from the tank or fuel lines. Other major sources are gasoline stations, handlers, and transporters; industries that use solvents; and users of paint and dry-cleaning fluids. Some hydrocarbons are known carcinogens; others play an important role in the formation of photochemical smog.

Other Pollutants.   A number of other substances with adverse effects on human health are emitted into the atmosphere from a variety of sources. EPA has established standards for four: asbestos, mercury, beryllium, and vinyl chloride. It lists three others (arsenic, benzene, and radionuclides) as "potentially hazardous." Many other substances, such as cadmium, pesticides, and numerous chemicals, are emitted by various industrial sources and could be added to this list.

CHRONIC EXPOSURE TO LOW LEVELS OF AIR POLLUTION

The adverse effects of acute exposure to air-borne pollutants have been demonstrated by three sources of data: (1) animal experimentation, (2) experimentation on human volunteers, and (3) morbidity and mortality figures gathered during acute air pollution episodes. The effects on human populations of chronic, low-level exposure have been more difficult to demonstrate. Evidence for the effects has come from epidemiologic studies; most of these have been retrospective or retrospective-cohort studies and have suffered from a number of problems. These include the difficulty of documenting exposure levels in a given population over a long period of time, the problems associated with identifying a nonexposed control group that is comparable to the exposed population under study, and the complexities of distinguishing the effects of ambient air pollution from those of concurrent exposures such as cigarette smoking and occupational exposures. Nonetheless, a host of studies have been reported during the past 30 years which, taken together, establish fairly conclusively a link between chronic low-level exposure to air-borne pollutants and a number of identifiable chronic illnesses. Among the conditions associated with air pollution are chronic obstructive pulmonary disease, bronchial asthma, cardiovascular disease, and acute respiratory disease. Associations between air pollution and both morbidity and mortality rates have been shown.

Mortality Rates and Air Pollution

One set of epidemiologic models that demonstrates the hazard to human health of air pollution focuses on correlations between levels of air-borne pollutants and mortality rates (from all causes). One of these models analyzes the changes in short-term mortality rates and correlates them with short-term changes in air pollution levels. This approach is well illustrated by a study by Buechley, Riggan, Hasselblad, and Van Bruggen (1973), of mortality rates in the New York metropolitan area. They demonstrated that on high-pollution days (SO_2 levels 1000 to 1300 $\mu g/m^3$), mortality rates averaged 2 percent more than expected, while on low-pollution days (SO_2 levels less than 30 $\mu g/m^3$), mortality rates averaged 1.5 percent less than expected. Between these two extremes, the relationship between mortality rates and SO_2 levels was almost linear.

An alternative approach is to study comparative long-term mortality rates in cities or communities with different levels of air pollution. A number of studies have been conducted using variations on this model and, in general, the data show a trend toward higher mortality rates in more polluted communities. A variety of methodological difficulties, however, prevent clear-cut interpretation of these reports (American Thoracic Society, 1978).

The weakness in epidemiologic studies that use overall mortality rates as an index of the impact of air pollution on health is that they fail to demonstrate a link between pollution and a given illness or set of illnesses. Other studies, however, have correlated pollution levels with specific diseases.

Air Pollution and Chronic Obstructive Pulmonary Disease

A variety of chronic respiratory conditions, including emphysema and chronic bronchitis, are classified as chronic obstructive pulmonary disease (COPD). Epidemiologic studies of the relationship between air pollution and COPD date back at least to 1958, when Fairbairn and Reid demonstrated a difference in the rates of sick leave, premature retirement, and death due to chronic bronchitis and pneumonia between British postal workers living in areas of high pollution and those living in areas of low pollution. Since then, over a score of reports have demonstrated similar relationships (American Thoracic Society, 1978). Populations in Britain, western Europe, Canada, the United States, and Japan have been studied; many of the studies have adjusted morbidity rates for age, sex, smoking habits, and occupation. Most of these reports have compared morbidity rates from COPD and related conditions between residents of more polluted and less polluted areas. When specific pollutants were studied, the sulfur dioxide/particulate complex was implicated most often.

An incompletely answered question regarding COPD and air pollution concerns the extent to which exposure to pollution causes the disease, as opposed to merely exacerbating preexisting disease. It is clear that there are causes of COPD other than air pollution. Cigarette smoking is the leading culprit; it also is known that some persons are genetically predisposed. Bates (1972) has proposed a model that outlines the mechanism by which suspended particulates act in concert with pollutant gases (SO_2, NO_2, and O_3) to damage the lung and produce emphysematous changes. However, it also is apparent from studies correlating short-term morbidity and mortality from COPD with short-term changes in pollution levels that airborne pollution does cause acute exacerbations of preexisting disease (Ciocco & Thompson, 1961; Lawther, Waller, & Henderson, 1970). Air pollution thus has been implicated as both a cause of COPD and a factor in acute exacerbations, although it is wholly responsible for neither.

Air Pollution and Bronchial Asthma

Bronchial asthma, although a chronic disease, is characterized by asymptomatic periods interrupted by acute attacks of variable frequency, intensity, and duration. The attacks typically consist of the rapid onset of bronchoconstriction and wheezing and may be mild or be severe enough to result in hospitalization and/or death.

Asthma most often is related to allergy, but increased levels of air pollution can precipitate acute attacks. One of the earliest reports on this phenomenon was a retrospective study of the Donora episode, which found that 87.6 percent of asthmatics stated that they had experienced symptoms (Schrenk et al., 1949). Numerous subsequent studies have demonstrated an association between increased pollution levels and an increased incidence of acute asthmatic attacks (Whittemore & Korn, 1980). Generally, these studies have used self-reported symptoms or emergency room visits as markers of asthma activity and have compared low-pollution with high-pollution days in a single location (rather than comparing two different populations).

No single pollutant has been implicated as the primary precipitant of acute asthmatic attacks. Moreover, a number of other factors have been found to be associated with an increased incidence of attacks, including season of the year, temperature, humidity, and even day of the week.

Air Pollution and Acute Respiratory Infections

In addition to evidence linking air pollution and chronic non-infectious disease, a number of studies demonstrate a relationship between exposure to air-borne pollutants and acute episodes of infectious respiratory disease (American Thoracic Society, 1978). Presumably, this relationship would be due to a pollutant-caused impairment of resistance to respiratory infection. Such an effect has been shown in animal models for SO_2, NO_2, and ozone.

The link between air pollution and infectious respiratory disease has been shown for both adults and children. In both age groups, increased air pollution is associated with an increase in lower-respiratory infection (pneumonia and bronchitis), but the association with upper-respiratory infection (colds and pharyngitis) is less clear. Two epidemiologic models have been used widely. One has shown an increased incidence of acute respiratory tract infections among persons living in more-polluted communities as compared to those living in less-polluted communities (Durham, 1974; Hammer, Miller, Stead, & Hayes, 1976). The other has demonstrated that, in a given community, the incidence of acute respiratory infections is greater during periods of increased air pollution (Levy, Gent, & Newhouse, 1977).

Air Pollution and Cardiovascular Disease

While air-borne pollutants are not thought to cause cardiovascular disease, it is apparent that air pollution causes exacerbation of symptoms and even death in persons with impaired coronary circulation. Carbon monoxide is the primary culprit. Aronow and Isbell (1973) demonstrated its ability to precipitate attacks of angina pectoris; the National Academy of Sciences (1974) estimated that 4000 deaths occur prematurely in the United States each year as a result of the exposure of persons with coronary artery disease to automobile exhaust.

Air Pollution and Lung Cancer

The role of air pollution as a factor in lung cancer etiology remains unclear. Cigarette smoking generally is acknowledged to be the primary cause of lung cancer; occupational exposures also play a role. There is, however, evidence that ambient air pollution also may be a factor. For instance, the incidence of lung cancer in urban areas is higher than that in rural areas (Haenszel, Loveland, & Sirken, 1962). Certain known carcinogens, particularly benzo(a)pyrene, are among the hydrocarbons found in polluted air (World Health Organization, 1972), and this substance has been implicated particularly as an ambient pulmonary carcinogen (Carnow & Meier, 1973; Menck, Casagrande, & Henderson, 1974).

Other epidemiologic studies designed to delineate more precisely the impact of air pollution on lung cancer rates have yielded conflicting results, and the subject remains controversial (American Thoracic Society, 1978).

Other Effects of Air Pollution

Air pollutants in industrial communities may reflect the by-products of the local industries and may present special health hazards. Smelters, for instance, may produce high levels of air-borne lead, and residents of the surrounding community may suffer demonstrable neurological damage as a result (Landrigan et al., 1976). Various industries may emit other heavy metals, asbestos, hydrocarbons, or radionuclides.

In addition to adverse health effects, air pollution may have a considerable nuisance value. Irritation to the eyes and mucous membranes is noticeable in many communities on high-pollution days; ozone is often the chief culprit. Objectionable odors also may be a problem, particularly in industrial areas.

Nonhealth-related economic damage caused by air-borne pollutants is an issue in many communities. "Acid rain," or acid deposition, has received considerable attention in recent years. The terms refer to complex processes in which air-borne sulfur oxides and nitrogen oxides interact with water vapor and sunlight to produce sulfuric acid (H_2SO_4) and nitric acid (HNO_3). These caustic substances then are deposited on the ground as aerosols or particulates or in rain, fog, dew, or snow (Council on Environmental Quality, 1982). In some areas, particularly in the Northeast, acid rain has been said to have caused significant crop and forest damage and to have rendered some lakes uninhabitable by fish. In response, the Acid Precipitation Act of 1980 established an Interagency Task Force to research the causes and effects of acid precipitation.

INDOOR AIR POLLUTION

In recent years, attention has focused increasingly on the quality of indoor air. Air pollutants found indoors may be the same as those simultaneously found outdoors, or these pollutants may be reduced, depending on the ventilation system of the building in question.

At the same time, pollutants may be produced inside dwellings, and these may render the indoor air considerably more hazardous than the air outside. The health effects of indoor air pollution recently have drawn the attention of the World Health Organization (Van Der Lende, 1980), the National Academy of Sciences (1981), and others.

Indoor air pollution may be a particularly important health problem for several reasons (Hinkle & Murray, 1981): (1) many people spend most of their lives indoors and may spend large amounts of time in the same room; (2) indoor air is enclosed, so substances emitted into it may reach high concentrations; (3) many normal indoor activities (cooking, cleaning, smoking) may release hazardous substances into the air; and (4) the materials of which the building itself is made may release hazardous substances, either because of volatility or radioactivity, or as a result of combustion.

This discussion primarily takes into account air pollutants found in dwellings. Hazardous indoor air pollutants found in occupational settings are discussed in Chapter 6.

The five primary classes of indoor air pollutants are:

1. *Infectious agents.* Although air-borne viruses and bacteria often are considered not to be an environmental health problem (Chapter 1), they are treated by many authors as indoor air pollutants. This is because they may be more concentrated in indoor than outdoor air, so the chances of transmission are accordingly greater indoors. Indeed, morbidity and mortality from influenza and pneumonia are greater during the winter months, when people spend more time indoors.

2. *Allergens.* "Natural pollutants" such as mold spores, danders, and dusts may occur in greater concentrations indoors than outdoors. Household items such as rugs and draperies serve as reservoirs for particulates such as these. Discarded or forgotten food items are sources of mold.

3. *Products of combustion.* Annually, approximately 4000 deaths and 63,000 disabling illnesses in the United States are caused by inhalation of combustion products indoors (Hinkle & Murray, 1981). Most of the deaths are the result of fires in buildings; approximately 80 percent of fire-related deaths are the result of inhalation of toxic gases (chiefly carbon monoxide), rather than the result of burns or other fire-related causes.

Toxic levels of carbon monoxide also may be created by the use of stoves, space heaters, or other appliances, or by automobiles in garages. These devices may be faulty or may be vented improperly. Other hazardous gases also may be produced, particularly NO_2 from gas stoves (Goldstein, Melia, & Florey, 1981).

Passive cigarette smoking has been recognized recently as a health hazard. Cigarette smoke may irritate the mucous membranes and/or cause allergic reactions in nonsmokers in the room. It also has been reported that the nonsmoking wives of heavy smokers may be at increased risk of lung cancer (Repace, 1981).

4. *Household products.* The indoor use of cleaning fluids, paint thinners, glues, and other volatile organic substances, particularly with inadequate ventilation, can lead to toxic concentrations of their vapors.

5. *Building materials.* Dwellings may include materials in their construction that are potentially hazardous. These include asbestos used to insulate heating ducts; radioactive radon contained in stone;

and particle board and urea foam insulation, which emit formaldehyde.

Although the hazards of many indoor air pollutants are well
recognized, there is a scarcity of relevant epidemiologic data available; hence, the magnitude of the problem of indoor air pollution
presently is not well defined. It may prove ultimately to be as serious a problem as the more well-studied outdoor air pollution.

PREVENTION OF AIR POLLUTION AND ASSOCIATED DISEASES

Reducing the level of air-borne pollutants is essential to a program of both primary and secondary prevention of certain conditions, as is evident from the previous discussion of health effects.
Clean rather than polluted air will prevent the development of significant numbers of cases of chronic obstructive pulmonary disease
and possibly cancer (primary prevention). It also will prevent morbidity and mortality in many preexisting cases of chronic obstructive pulmonary disease, bronchial asthma, coronary artery disease,
and other conditions (secondary prevention).

As discussed previously, the EPA has set National Ambient
Air Quality Standards (NAAQS). Among other things, these standards established emission limitations for new pollutant sources, such
as new factories and automobiles. States must use these new-source
limitations and their own regulation of existing sources to attain the
NAAQS; their strategies for doing so are to be spelled out in State
Implementation Plans (see Chapter 8).

National Ambient Air Quality Standards are shown in Table
5-1 (see p. 127). Primary standards are based on the level required
to protect the public health; secondary standards represent the level
necessary to protect the "public welfare"—crops, painted surfaces,
and the like.

Air quality is monitored by a variety of devices at over 7000
stations across the United States. Most of these are operated by state
or local pollution control agencies. The technology for measuring
the concentration of air-borne pollutants is constantly improving.
The values obtained at a given sampling station depend on the lo-

cation of the station relative to sources of pollution, the method used to measure pollutant concentrations, and other factors. The EPA has published standards for such stations and, in reporting national data on air pollution, uses information gathered from varying numbers of sites ranging from fewer than 400 for CO to over 2600 for total suspended particulates (Council on Environmental Quality, 1982).

Presently, air quality in metropolitan areas is evaluated according to the Pollutant Standards Index (PSI), which was developed by the EPA, the Council on Environmental Quality, and the Department of Commerce (Federal Interagency Task Force, 1976). This is shown in Table 5-3. The formula for the PSI takes into account five of the seven criteria pollutants (all except hydrocarbons and lead) and will yield a value of 100 or more ("unhealthful") if the concentration of any one of these pollutants rises to the level of its primary air quality standard at any monitoring station in the metropolitan area. Air quality is deemed "good" (PSI less than 50) only when ambient concentrations of all five pollutants are less than half the primary standards at all monitoring stations. Index values are often reported by the media to enable persons with chronic respiratory or cardiac disease to respond to dangerously high levels of pollution.

Monitoring of pollution levels in recent years has demonstrated a steady improvement in air quality in metropolitan areas, most of it attributed to the surveillance, regulation, and enforcement called for by the Clean Air Act and its amendments. For instance, combined data from 23 such areas show that the average number of days in which the PSI exceeded 100 declined from 87 in 1974 to 58 in 1980, while the average number of days in which it exceeded 200 declined from 23 to 15 (Council on Environmental Quality, 1982). Air pollution remains a major problem in many metropolitan areas, however. Between 1978 and 1980, six cities averaged over 100 days per year of PSI readings above 100. Los Angeles averaged 231 such days per year (Council on Environmental Quality, 1979); an average of 113 days per year in Los Angeles had a PSI over 200. In 1980, 508 United States counties were classified officially as not in attainment with EPA standards for ozone; 379 were not in attainment for particulates; 163 for CO; 95 for SO_2; 21 for lead; and seven for NO_2 (Council on Environmental Quality, 1982).

With respect to total pollutant emissions, Table 5-4 shows that

Table 5-3 Pollutant Standards Index (PSI) and Health Effects Associated with the Various Levels

PSI value	Descriptor	Health Effects	Warning
400 and above	Hazardous	Premature death of ill and elderly. Healthy people will experience adverse symptoms that affect their normal activity.	All persons should remain indoors, keeping windows and doors closed. All persons should minimize physical exertion and avoid traffic.
300–399	Hazardous	Premature onset of certain diseases in addition to significant aggravation of symptoms and decreased exercise tolerance in healthy persons.	Elderly and persons with existing diseases should stay indoors and avoid physical exertion. General population should avoid outdoor activity.
200–299	Very unhealthful	Significant aggravation of symptoms and decreased exercise tolerance in persons with heart or lung disease, with widespread symptoms in the healthy population.	Elderly and persons with existing heart or lung disease should stay indoors and reduce physical activity.
100–199	Unhealthful	Mild aggravation of symptoms in susceptible persons, with irritation symptoms in the healthy population.	Persons with existing heart or respiratory ailments should reduce physical exertion and outdoor activity.
50–99	Moderate		
0–49	Good		

Source: Council on Environmental Quality. *Environmental Quality 1981.* Washington, D.C.: U.S. Government Printing Office, 1982.

Table 5-4   National Air Pollutant Emissions, by Pollutant, 1940–1980
(millions of metric tons)

	1940	1950	1960	1970	1980
Particulates	21.9	23.2	20.2	17.6	7.8
Sulfur oxides	17.4	19.6	19.2	27.9	23.7
Nitrogen oxides	6.5	9.3	12.7	18.5	20.7
Hydrocarbons	13.9	17.5	21.6	27.1	21.8
Carbon monoxide	74.7	82.8	90.8	110.9	85.4

Source: Council on Environmental Quality. *Environmental Quality 1981*. Washington, D.C.:
U.S. Government Printing Office, 1982.

a worsening situation has been generally reversed since 1970. In particular, significant strides have been made in the reduction of total suspended particulates. The amount of nitrogen oxides emitted continues to increase, however.

In general, longitudinal data are not available for documenting changes in health status that may correspond to these secular trends in air quality. Information from the National Health and Nutrition Examination Survey (NHANES), however, does demonstrate a nationwide decrease in average blood lead levels paralleling reduced lead emissions from automobiles between 1976 and 1980 (*Morbidity and Mortality Weekly Report*, 1982).

Two approaches generally have been used in attempting to reduce air pollution. The first is to reduce the production of pollutants, for instance, by using cleaner fuels. The second is to limit pollutant emissions through the use of devices such as scrubbers and electrostatic precipitators. Coal-fired steam electric generating plants have turned to coal with lower sulfur levels; in addition, EPA standards require all new plants to remove 85 percent of potential SO_2 emissions, regardless of the sulfur level of the coal used, through the use of scrubbers. These are devices that use limestone (calcium carbonate) or nahcolite (sodium bicarbonate) to absorb gaseous sulfates.

Electrostatic precipitators are installed on stacks to control particulate output and may reduce such emissions by 90 to 99 percent. Other devices used to control industrial emissions include gravitational and cyclone collectors, filters, and afterburners (United States

DHEW, 1969). Emissions of NO_2 from stationary sources have been reduced by the installation of more efficient equipment and by precise adjustments of flames and air flows on present equipment (Council on Environmental Quality, 1982). Hydrocarbon emissions have been reduced in part by controlling the evaporation of volatile fuels and chemicals and by reducing leaks and venting.

Transportation, however, remains the largest single source of air pollutants. Most cars produced in the United States since 1975 have used catalytic converters to meet new-source emission standards, particularly for NO_2, CO, and ozone. Some smaller cars have used electronic fuel injection techniques to achieve the same result. Diesel engines have gained in popularity but, while these meet standards for criteria pollutants, they emit carcinogenic carbon compounds (Council on Environmental Quality, 1980). In some locations, however, advances in engine technology may be inadequate to achieve acceptable levels of air quality. Reduction in automobile use, with substitution of urban rail systems or other alternative means of transportation, may be required. Like many other issues in environmental health, this ultimately may be a social or political issue, rather than a question of technology or medicine.

REFERENCES

American Thoracic Society (1978). *Health Effects of Air Pollution*. New York: American Lung Association.

Aronow WS, and Isbell, NW (1973). Carbon Monoxide Effect on Exercise-Induced Angina Pectoris. *Ann Intern Med 79*:392–395.

Bates DV (1972). Air Pollutants and the Human Lung. *Amer Rev Resp Dis 105*: 1–13.

Buechley RW, Riggan WB, Hasselblad V, and Van Bruggen JB (1973). SO_2 Levels and Perturbations in Mortality. A Study in the New York–New Jersey Metropolis. *Arch Environ Health 27*:134–137.

Carnow VW, and Meier P (1973). Air Pollution and Pulmonary Cancer. *Arch Environ Health 27*:207–218.

Ciocco A, and Thompson DJ (1961). A Follow-up of Donora Ten Years After: Methodology and Findings. *Am J Pub Health 51*:155–164.

Corman R (1978). *Air Pollution Primer*. New York: American Lung Association.

Council on Environmental Quality (1971). *Environmental Quality 1970*. Washington, D.C.: U.S. Government Printing Office.

Council on Environmental Quality (1980). *Environmental Quality 1979*. Washington, D.C.: U.S. Government Printing Office.

Council on Environmental Quality (1982). *Environmental Quality 1981*. Washington, D.C.: U.S. Government Printing Office.

Durham WH (1974). Air Pollution and Student Health. *Arch Environ Health* 28:241-254.

Fairbairn AS, and Reid DD (1958). Air Pollution and Other Local Factors in Respiratory Disease. *Br J Prev Soc Med 12*:94-103.

Federal Interagency Task Force on Air Quality Indicators (1976). *A Recommended Air Pollution Index*. Washington, D.C.: U.S. Government Printing Office.

Firket J (1931). The Cause of the Symptoms Found in the Meuse Valley during the Fog of December 1930. *Bull R Acad Med 11*:683.

Freeman G, Juhos LT, Furiosi HN, Mussenden R, Stephes RJ, and Evans MJ (1974). Pathology of Pulmonary Disease from Exposure to Interdependent Ambient Gases (NO_2 and O_3). *Arch Environ Health 29*:203-210.

Freeman G, Stephes RJ, Crane SC, and Furiosi NJ (1968). Lesion of the Lung in Rats Continuously Exposed to Two Parts Per Million of Nitrogen Dioxide. *Arch Environ Health 17*:181-192.

Goldstein BD, Melia RJW, and Florey CDV (1981). Indoor Nitrogen Oxides. *Bull NY Acad Med 57*:873-879.

Greenburg L, Jacobs MB, Drolette BM, Field F, and Braverman MM (1963). Report of an Air Pollution Incident in New York City, November 1953. *Public Health Reports 78*:1061-1064.

Hackney HD, Linn WS, Karuza SK, Buckley RD, Law DC, Bates DV, Jazucha M, Pengelly LD, and Silverman F (1977). Effects of Ozone Exposure in Canadians and Southern Californians. *Arch Environ Health 32*:110-116.

Haenszel W, Loveland DB, and Sirken MG (1962). Lung Cancer Mortality as Related to Residence and Smoking Histories: I. White Males. *J Nat Cancer Inst 28*:947-1001.

Hammer DI, Miller FJ, Stead AG, and Hayes CG (1976). Air Pollution and Child Lower Respiratory Disease. I. Exposure to Sulfur Oxides and Particulate Matter in New York, 1972. In AJ Finkel and WC Duel (eds.) *Clinical Implications of Air Pollution Research*. Acton, Mass.: Publishing Sciences Group.

Hinkle LE, and Murray SH (1981). The Importance of the Quality of Indoor Air. *Bull NY Acad Med 57*:827-872.

Landrigan PJ, Baker EL, Feldman RG, Cox DH, Eden RV, Ornstein WA, Mather JA, Jankel AJ, and Von Lindern SH (1976): Increased Lead Absorption with Anemia and Slower Nerve Conduction in Children Near a Lead Smelter. *J Pediatr 89*:904-910.

Lawther PJ, Waller RE, and Henderson M (1970). Air Pollution and Exacerbations of Bronchitis. *Thorax 25*:525-539.

Levy D, Gent M, and Newhouse MT (1977). Relationship between Acute Respiratory Illness and Air Pollution Levels in an Industrial City. *Am Rev Respir Dis 116*:167-173.

Logan WPD (1953). Mortality in London Fog Incident. *Lancet 1*:336-338.

McCarroll J, and Bradley W (1966). Excess Mortality as an Indicator of Health Effects of Air Pollution. *Am J Pub Health 56*:1933-1942.

Melia RJW, Florey C, Altman DG, and Swan AV (1977). Association between Gas Cooking and Respiratory Disease in Children. *Br Med J 2*:149-152.

Menck, HR, Casagrande JT, and Henderson BE (1974). Industrial Air Pollution: Possible Effect on Lung Cancer. *Science 183*:210-212.

Morbidity and Mortality Weekly Report (1982). Blood Lead Levels in US Population. *31*:132-134.

National Academy of Sciences — National Academy of Engineering (1974). *Air Quality and Automobile Emission Control. Vol. 2: Health Effects of Air Pollutants.* Committee on Public Works, U.S. Senate, no. 93-24. Washington, D.C.: U.S. Government Printing Office.

National Academy of Sciences (1981). *Indoor Pollutants.* Washington, D.C.: National Academy Press.

Orehek J, Massari JP, Garrard P, Gremaud C, and Charpin J (1976). Effect of Short-Term, Low Level Nitrogen Dioxide Exposure on Bronchial Sensitivity of Asthmatic Patients. *J Clin Invest 57*:301-307.

Repace JL (1981). The Problem of Passive Smoking. *Bull NY Acad Med 57*: 936-961.

Schrenk HH, Heimann H, Clayton GD, Gafafer W, and Wexler H (1949). Air Pollution in Donora, Pennsylvania. Epidemiology of the Unusual Smog Episode of October 1948. *Public Health Bulletin 306*, U.S. Government Printing Office, Washington, D.C.

Scott JA (1963). The London Fog Incident of December 1962. *Med Officer 109*:250.

U.S. DHEW (1969). Control Techniques for Particulate Air Pollutants. Washington, D.C.: U.S. Public Health Service, publication no. AP-51.

Van Der Lende R (1980). Health Aspects Related to Indoor Air Pollution. *International J Epidemiol 9*:195-197.

Weir FW, and Bromberg PA (1972). Further Investigation of the Effects of Sulfur Dioxide on Human Subjects. Washington, D.C.: American Petroleum Institute, projects no. CAWC S-15.

Whittemore AS, and Korn EL (1980). Asthma and Air Pollution in the Los Angeles Area. *Am J Pub Health 70*:687-696.

World Health Organization (1972). Health Hazards of the Human Environment. Geneva: World Health Organization.

Chapter 6

Occupational Health

James M. Melius*
Philip J. Landrigan

Occupationally related injuries and illnesses are an important public health problem in this country. Each year approximately one of every 11 American workers suffers an illness or injury due to hazardous exposures in the work environment (Bureau of Labor Statistics, 1980). Approximately 4500 job-related deaths and 5.5 million job-related injuries occur in workplaces with 11 or more employees. These injuries lead to over 38 million lost workdays. Accurate information on diseases and deaths due to occupational exposure is more difficult to obtain. An estimate made in the early 1970s projected an annual incidence of approximately 100,000 deaths and 400,000 illnesses due to occupational disease (*President's Report*, 1972).

Although recognition of the effects on health of occupational exposures dates back to at least 2000 B.C., and many occupational diseases were well recognized in medieval times, the major epidemics of occupational disease that have occurred since the Industrial Revolution are responsible for much of our current recognition of the

---

*This chapter was written by James M. Melius and Philip J. Landrigan as part of their activities while in the employment of the U.S. Department of Health and Human Services.

importance of the work environment to health. These epidemics of occupational disease include:

1. *Coal workers' pneumonoconiosis*. Although the occurrence of coal workers' pneumonoconiosis was recognized in England in the 1800s, very little attention was paid to the disease in the United States until the 1960s. A Public Health Service study of coal miners in the 1960s found that 11 percent of Appalachian coal miners had radiographic evidence of pneumonoconiosis (Lainhart, 1971). This study and other similar findings eventually led to the passage of the Federal Coal Mine Health and Safety Act of 1969.

2. *Gauley Bridge*. In the 1930s, an estimated 470 men died and 1500 were disabled due to silicosis from exposure while building a hydroelectric tunnel near Gauley Bridge, West Virginia (House Committee on Labor, 1936).

3. *Bladder cancer in the dye industry*. Although a high incidence of bladder cancer in dye manufacturing workers was first recognized in Switzerland in 1875 (Rehn, 1875), the magnitude of the problem was not recognized until 1942 when Hueper showed that the development of the chemical dye industry in a number of countries was followed up to 30 years later by an epidemic of urinary bladder cancers among the exposed workers (Hueper, 1942).

4. *Kepone and neurological diseases*. In 1975, an investigation at a chemical plant in Virginia found that 73 of 114 production workers exposed in the manufacturing of a pesticide, Kepone, had evidence of nervous system damage (Cannon, Veazey, Jackson, et al., 1978). The chief manifestations of the neurological damage were tremors, visual difficulties, a feeling of nervousness, and personality changes. Other recent epidemics of occupational neurological disease have resulted from exposure to methyl butyl ketone (Billmaier, Allen, Craft, et al., 1974), n-hexane (Herskowitz, Ishii, & Schaumburg, 1971), and dimethylaminoproprionitrile (Kreiss, Wegman, Niles, et al., 1980).

5. *Asbestos*. Although the occupational health hazards of asbestos exposure have been well recognized for many years, from World War II to the 1960s between 8 and 11 million workers were exposed to the material in shipyards. Epidemiological studies of workers exposed to asbestos have found that approximately one-half of them died

from asbestos-related lung disease or cancer (Selikoff, 1978). A National Institute for Occupational Safety and Health (NIOSH) study, conducted in the early 1970s, estimated that 1.6 million workers were being exposed to asbestos at that time (NIOSH, 1977a).

    6. *DBCP and male infertility.* In July 1977, a study conducted by NIOSH at an agricultural chemical plant in California found that 32 workers exposed to DBCP, an agricultural nematocide, had low sperm counts due to this exposure (Whorton, Milby, & Krauss, et al., 1979). Fourteen of these workers were azoospermic. Twelve of the azoospermic workers were reexamined one year later, and all were still azoospermic, suggesting probable irreversible testicular dysfunction (Whorton & Milby, 1980). This investigation was initiated when several workers noted that they were having difficulty fathering children.

    Workplace tragedies where many workers have died due to fires or other safety hazards also have been important in drawing attention to occupational safety and health:

- In 1907, the worst mine disaster in United States history took 361 lives in Monongah, West Virginia.
- In 1911, a fire at the Triangle Shirt Waist Company in New York City killed 146 workers, mostly young women.
- In 1968, a coal mine exploded in Farmington, West Virginia, killing 78 miners.
- In 1978, a massive scaffolding on a concrete cooling tower at Willow Island, West Virginia collapsed, killing 51 construction workers.

    Today, a major focus of occupational health practice is the prevention of future epidemics that might result from the introduction of new toxic materials and processes. New and growing industries such as synthetic fiber products, the electronics industry, and biotechnological production involve possibly-unrecognized hazards from these new work environments. Information on the toxic effects of current occupational exposure is evolving rapidly, necessitating new measures to protect the health of workers exposed in these industries.

SOCIAL AND POLITICAL FACTORS IN THE PREVENTION OF OCCUPATIONAL DISEASE AND INJURY

All occupational disease is of human origin; therefore, it should be highly amenable to prevention. The immediate costs of reducing exposure may be quite high, however, and therefore resisted by industry. The benefits of regulation are delayed and usually not easily discernible in economic terms. For these reasons, political action has been important in achieving prevention of occupational illnesses and injuries.

Legislation

Before 1970, most regulations pertaining to occupational safety and health were established by state governments and varied widely across the country (Nothstein, 1981). Increased interest in occupational safety and health and the deficiencies of the state-based system of regulation led to the passage of the Occupational Safety and Health Act of 1970. (The act is discussed in detail in the appendix to this chapter.) This act established the Occupational Safety and Health Administration (OSHA), whose task is to set occupational safety and health standards and to enforce them. Although state governments still could be involved in regulation and enforcement, their actions were to be at least as effective as OSHA's.

The act also established the National Institute for Occupational Safety and Health (NIOSH), whose task is to perform occupational safety and health research, to develop criteria for standards, and to help train occupational safety and health professionals.

Although OSHA has improved the regulation of the occupational environment greatly, its effectiveness has been hampered by political opposition, by lack of funding for enforcement, and by long legal challenges to new regulations. As a result of the latter, relatively few new regulations have been implemented. Most current regulations are "consensus" standards adopted by OSHA from outside groups (e.g., the American Conference of Governmental Industrial Hygienists) in the early 1970s.

In 1977, the Mine Safety and Health Acts Amendments were

passed by Congress. These amendments consolidated federal regulation of occupational safety and health in mining under the administration of one group, the Mine Safety and Health Administration (MSHA) and strengthened the legislative basis for mining regulation and enforcement. Although regulation and enforcement have always been stronger for mining than for general industry (due to the greater risks in mining), MSHA has had many of the same problems as OSHA.

Workers' Compensation

In the early 1900s, most states adopted workers' compensation laws. These laws were intended to protect industry from liability suits due to occupational diseases and injuries and at the same time to protect disabled workers and their families from the delays and costs involved in legal action. Under these laws, an injured or disabled worker would be compensated at a predetermined rate for a given injury or illness, depending on the degree of disability. In return, the worker could not sue the employer for any further liability. The costs would be covered by insurance purchased by the company to compensate such workers.

Unfortunately, this system does not work as well as intended, for several reasons. There is much state-to-state variation in benefits and requirements for compensation. Maintaining low insurance rates by limiting those compensated often is seen as a way to attract industry to a state. In most states, benefits are quite low and usually do not compensate a worker fully for the injury or illness and for the time lost from work.

While injury decisions are usually straightforward, compensation for occupational diseases is usually poor, due to outdated definitions of compensable diseases, unavailability of exposure information, and inadequate consideration of disease latency. A recent study found that fewer than 10 percent of occupational disease cases are compensated by workers' compensation (U.S. Department of Labor, 1980). Most cases already receive benefits from the Social Security Disability Program or other government programs in which costs are borne by the general public rather than by the responsible industries.

Due to the defects of the present compensation system, liability suits against equipment and chemical suppliers (which are allowed in some states) are being used more often in place of workers' compensation. For instance, in the case of asbestos-related diseases, millions of dollars in suits have been brought against asbestos suppliers. Legislative consideration is being given now to proposals to develop a national workers' compensation system and to limit third-party or product-liability suits. There is a precedent in that coal workers' pneumoconiosis was so prevalent that federal legislation was enacted to help compensate these workers and to administer the compensation program.

Other Groups Involved

The increasing focus on occupational safety and health has led to increased efforts by many groups to reduce work-related injuries or illnesses, among them, industry, unions, universities, and state governments.

Industry.   Due to the increased recognition of the need for better safety and health programs and to increased pressure from workers, unions, and the government, industry recently has improved greatly its efforts in occupational safety and health. This effort has led to the development of improved safety and health programs and to greater research efforts in the toxicology of industrial products and in occupational health.

Unions.   Unions have always recognized the need for greater attention to occupational safety and health to protect their membership. Most large international unions have occupational safety and health staffs who train and provide information to their membership, help negotiate health and safety provisions in their contracts, and help press for better regulation and enforcement.

Universities.   Many universities have initiated or expanded programs for training occupational health and safety professionals and conducting research in this field.

State Governments.   Despite federal control of regulations and their enforcement, many state governments, through their health or labor departments, still are involved in enforcement activities (under the guidance of OSHA and MSHA) and in consultations on health and safety for private industry (particularly small businesses).

Some also are developing research programs in occupational and environmental health.

PREVENTIVE MEASURES

Exposure Criteria

The standard approach for preventing occupational health effects has been to determine an exposure level below which nearly all exposed workers will not develop adverse health effects, and then to maintain exposures below that level. These exposure criteria may be developed for chronic effects and be set for the usual workday, or they may be developed as ceiling levels for short-term exposures to prevent acute health effects. The criteria for setting standards usually are based on epidemiological studies, medical studies, and/or animal testing.

Many occupational exposure standards have been established in the United States by OSHA and MSHA; however, other non-regulatory groups commonly develop exposure criteria, too. These groups include NIOSH, the American Conference of Governmental Industrial Hygienists (ACGIH), and industrial associations. Criteria regarding occupational safety also are developed by a variety of groups and by the regulatory agencies. These criteria may specify equipment design, load requirements, protective devices, and performance requirements.

Preventive Measures for Occupational Exposures

Several methods may be used to control occupational exposure and prevent occupational injury or illness. Whenever feasible, a less-toxic substance should be substituted for a more-toxic substance in an industrial process. Changes in the design of industrial equipment (e.g., vibrating hand tools) may be undertaken to reduce exposures or to prevent injuries. Enclosing an industrial process is an example of a common approach taken to reduce chemical or noise exposures. Exposures also may be reduced by local exhaust ventilation or general room ventilation. In addition, proper work practices are an important method for reducing exposures and helping to prevent accidents. Educating workers and their supervisors to the danger of occupational exposures and to proper practices for controlling exposures is essential. Personal protective equipment (respirators, hearing protection, etc.) should be used only if engineering controls or work practice controls for reducing or preventing exposures are not feasible. Proper design, fitting, and use are required for this equipment to be effective; however, compliance with use may be a problem. Initially, medical screening may be used to identify individuals unfit for a particular job or unusually susceptible to a specific exposure. Screening also may be done to detect early signs of occupational illness and thus prevent further progression of illness due to continued exposure. Unfortunately, most occupational medical screening programs have not been critically evaluated in regard to their effectiveness.

OCCUPATIONAL HAZARDS

As part of their jobs today, many workers are exposed to hazards that range from chronic trauma and pesticide exposures to psychological stress.

Safety Hazards

The risk of injury in the workplace varies with the job. Table 6–1 shows the 10 industries with the highest injury incidence rates in 1978. These rates range from 24.3 per 100 full-time workers in the special products sawmill industry to 13.5 in the steel springs industry.

In 1978, four of 10 job-related fatalities were associated with the operation of motor vehicles and industrial vehicles and equipment (Bureau of Labor Statistics, 1980). Falls accounted for 13 percent of the deaths, and electrocutions 7 percent.

The causes of industrial accidents involve multiple factors that vary with the industry and the type of work. Two main approaches to the causes of accidents have developed. One tries to explain accidents in terms of personal factors such as "accident prone" (Chambers & Yule, 1941), while the other has concentrated on the etiologi-

Table 6-1   Ten Industries with the Highest Injury Incidence Rates, 1978

Industry	Rate[a]
Special products sawmills	24.3
Reclaimed rubber	17.4
Malt	16.6
Logging camps and logging contractors	15.5
Mobile homes	15.1
Structured wood members	15.0
Sanitary services	15.0
Meatpacking plants	14.8
Vitreous plumbing fixtures	14.5
Steel springs	13.5

[a]Incidence rate of lost workday injuries per 100 full-time workers.

Source: Bureau of Labor Statistics. Occupational Injuries and Illnesses in the United States, by Industry, 1978. Washington, D.C.: U.S. Department of Labor, 1980.

cal characteristics in the environment, such as unguarded machines (Haddon, Suchman, & Klein, 1964). Clearly, both factors may be involved. Much current research is focusing on study methods evaluating both factors (Saari & Lahtela, 1981).

Chronic Trauma

Chronic trauma to the musculoskeletal system caused by repetitive motion or overexertion is a major source of morbidity and disability among workers in this country. Solid data on the overall incidence and prevalence of these musculoskeletal problems are not available; however, the National Safety Council estimates that 25 percent of all workplace injuries are attributable to overexertion associated with manual materials handling (NIOSH, 1981b). Low back pain, carpal tunnel syndrome (a type of musculoskeletal injury in the wrist), and problems in other joints account for most of the morbidity due to chronic trauma (Armstrong & Chaffin, 1979; Chaffin, 1975).

A variety of factors contributes to the development of chronic trauma problems, including lifting requirements, physical fitness, history of similar previous problems, posture required for the task, and repetition of movements. Much research has been done in the past several years to determine the contribution of these various factors and to develop guidelines for preventing the occurrence of these problems (Armstrong & Chaffin, 1979; NIOSH, 1981b; Wasserman, Badger, Doyle, & Margolies, 1974). (Obviously, these factors will vary from job to job, leading to different degrees of risk in different industries.

A related cause of occupational health problems is exposure to vibration, usually in the use of vibrating hand tools. Approximately 8 million workers in the United States are exposed to vibration from hand-held vibrating tools such as pneumatic drills and chain saws (NIOSH, 1981a). The most common medical problem due to vibration exposure is vibration white finger (VWF), a condition associated with cold-induced pallor of the fingers, which may progress to severe chronic disability. The prevalence of VWF in foundry workers using vibrating grinding tools has been found in one study to be 47 percent (NIOSH, 1977f). Similarly, high prevalences have been found in shipyard workers, pneumatic drill operators, and chain-saw operators. Control of these hazards is focused on redesigning tools to reduce their vibration forces.

Noise

Approximately 40 percent of American workers have significant exposure to noise in the workplace. Chronic exposure to high levels of noise may lead initially to hearing loss at higher noise frequencies. With continued exposure, this hearing deficit increases and expands to include lower frequencies (including those used in speech). Eventually, partial or complete deafness may result. Control of noise exposure is the primary means of prevention. Engineering changes or enclosure of the sources of noise may reduce noise exposure significantly. If engineering controls are not feasible, personal protective devices may be necessary. Routine audiometric screening of workers exposed to noise is also important in preventing serious hearing deficits.

Radiation

There are several major categories of occupational radiation exposure (NIOSH, 1977h). Workers may be exposed to ionizing radiation (particularly x-rays) from x-ray machines and from work in nuclear facilities. Although acute radiation illness is very rare in industry, long-term radiation exposure may cause various forms of cancer. Exposure to alpha radiation (from radon daughters; see Chapter 4) is a serious hazard for uranium and certain other miners, and a substantial risk of developing lung cancer has been found for these miners.

Ultraviolet light is a significant occupational exposure for outdoor workers, welders, and glass workers. The health effects induced by ultraviolet light exposure include skin irritation, severe eye irritation, and eventually skin cancer. Infrared light is a significant occupational exposure for workers in glassmaking, welding, steel, foundry, and related industries (NIOSH, 1982). Excessive exposures may lead to cataracts, skin burns, and eye burns. Lasers are used in industrial cutting operations, construction surveying, and medical treatment. Potential health effects of exposure to lasers include eye, skin, and tissue burns.

Workers exposed to microwaves include communication workers and radar operators, as well as workers near radio frequency heat sealers and other microwave drying equipment. The potential health effects from overexposure to microwaves include tissue burns and cataracts. Currently, there is concern about potential reproductive effects resulting from chronic exposure to microwaves.

Heavy Metals

Exposure to heavy metals is a major cause of occupational disease. In addition to lead, discussed in Chapters 3 and 5, some important heavy metal exposures include:

1. *Cadmium.* Exposure occurs in pigment workers, painters, and welders (Lee & White, 1980). Acute overexposure to cadmium fumes may cause pulmonary damage, while chronic exposure is as-

sociated with renal tubular damage and an increased risk of cancer of the prostate.

2. *Arsenic*. Exposure occurs in smelter workers, glassworkers, and pesticide workers (Landrigan, 1981). High exposures to arsenic may cause neurological damage, kidney damage, and dermatitis. Chronic exposure is associated with an increased risk of skin, lung, and liver cancer.

3. *Manganese*. Exposure occurs among welders and other metal workers (Tanaka, 1975). The health effects of overexposure to manganese include respiratory infections and neurological damage (a disease similar to Parkinson's disease).

Dusts

Health effects caused by dusts depend on the size of the particle (which determines how far it is carried into the respiratory tree), the body's reaction to the inhaled particulate matter, the possible absorption of the particulate matter into the body from the lung, and the local respiratory toxicity of the substance (Lemen & Dement, 1979).

Some inhaled dusts (e.g., asbestos, silica) may cause fibrosis or scarring of the lung tissue. Over a period of time, the fibrosis may be sufficient to affect pulmonary function severely, leading to significant respiratory disability. Other dusts may be irritating to the respiratory tract due to the chemical or physical properties of the dust (i.e., alkaline dusts). Over a period of time, these dusts may lead to the development of bronchitis. For some occupational dust exposures (usually organic dusts), an immunological reaction may develop and lead to respiratory disease (e.g., allergic alveolitis). Some dusts, most notably asbestos, are carcinogenic and greatly increase the risk of lung or other cancers among exposed workers.

Solvents

Solvents are used commonly in industry as cleaning solutions, as ingredients in paints and varnishes, and in organic chemical synthesis. Solvents have a variety of toxic effects (NIOSH, 1977a), including neurotoxicity, dermatological effects, carcinogenesis, reproductive effects, and other organ-specific toxicities. These effects are discussed in more detail later in the chapter.

Gases

Some gases may act as simple asphyxiants by displacing the oxygen in the atmosphere. Exposure to these gases usually causes health problems only if a person is working in a confined space without adequate outside ventilation. Other gases act as chemical asphyxiants by causing a metabolic change leading to asphyxiation. For example, carbon monoxide binds to hemoglobin, thus displacing oxygen molecules (NIOSH, 1977e).

Chlorine and oxides of nitrogen may cause irritation of the respiratory tract, leading to acute or chronic respiratory disease. Exposure to phosgene and other gases may cause a severe pulmonary irritation of delayed onset, which is often fatal. Exposure to some gases may cause toxicity to other organ systems. For example, arsine exposure may lead to hemolytic anemia. Exposure to nitrous oxide (used in anesthesia) is associated with an increased risk of birth defects and miscarriages in pregnant women (NIOSH, 1977e).

Organic Chemicals

Organic chemicals are important in occupational health because of their wide use (in paints, plastics, resins, etc.) and because they may be toxic at low levels of exposure. The following are a few examples:

1. *Vinyl chloride.* Mainly used to produce polyvinyl chloride, this is an important base for many plastics. Occupational exposure to the vinyl chloride monomer can lead to liver disease, vascular disease of the fingers, angiosarcoma (an otherwise rare cancer of the liver), and cancers of the lung and possibly of the brain (Falk, Creech, Heath, et al., 1974; Lloyd, 1975). (See Chapter 4.)

2. *Polychlorinated biphenyls* (PCBs). These are associated with liver disease, neuropathy, and chloracne (an acnelike skin dis-

ease). PCBs also are suspected of causing cancer and reproductive effects (Kimbrough, 1980). For a detailed discussion of PCBs, see Chapter 3.

3. *Dimethylamine propionitrite* (DMAPN). An organic resin catalyst, DMAPN has been found to cause a neuropathy mainly affecting the nerves supplying the bladder (Kreiss, et al., 1980).

4. *Bischloromethyl ether* (BCME). This organic chemical intermediate has been found to cause a high risk of lung cancer (Lemen, Johnson, Wagoner, et al., 1976).

Pesticides and Herbicides

Pesticides and herbicides are of particular significance because of the large number of agricultural and other workers exposed and because of the severe toxicity of many of these compounds (NIOSH, 1977g). The toxicity of Kepone® and DBCP was discussed earlier. A more common occupational health problem involves widespread exposure to pesticides that are cholinesterase inhibitors. These pesticides affect nerve impulse transmission, leading to a variety of acute symptoms (headaches, sweating, rapid heartbeat, muscle fasciculations). Other pesticides and herbicides may have more severe specific health effects; leptophos, for instance, causes neuropathy, and paraquat causes pulmonary fibrosis when inhaled.

Psychological Stress Factors

Although difficult to separate from other sources of psychological stress, work factors obviously play a role in the psychological well-being of most people. Work stress factors may contribute to the occurrence of psychological disease or symptoms, to the occurrence of other diseases (e.g., heart disease), and to other problems such as alcoholism and drug abuse. Much occupational health and psychological research currently is being done to improve understanding of the role of work-related stress factors and to develop methods for reducing these problems (NIOSH, 1978).

OCCUPATIONAL DISEASES

Recognized occupational diseases include acute and chronic illnesses of many organ systems. Many occupational diseases may become manifest only after years of exposure or many years after last exposure. Most are not specific occupational diseases but rather "common" diseases that may be caused by occupational exposures or other factors. In many cases, a combination of occupational exposures and other risk factors (e.g., cigarette smoking) may act together to cause the disease. For these reasons, occupational diseases are often very difficult to recognize as being related to occupational exposures. A thorough occupational history is essential to the medical evaluation of any patient, in determining whether or not that patient's disease may be related to the work environment.

Dermatitis

Occupational skin disease is the most prevalent type of occupational illness. Surveillance data for California indicate an incidence rate for occupational skin disease of 2.1 per 1000 workers per year, with much higher rates among workers in certain industries, particularly agricultural and chemical workers (California Department of Industrial Relations, 1982). Twenty percent of these affected workers lose time from work because of skin disease, for an average loss per affected worker of nine working days.

There are several major categories of occupational skin disease (NIOSH, 1977c). Irritant dermatitis may be caused by irritating compounds (including oils, solvents, some metals, etc.) that cause an inflammation of the exposed areas of skin. Workers also may become sensitized to certain compounds (nickel, platinum, epoxy resins, etc.), leading to a recurrent or chronic dermatitis unless the exposure is discontinued. Exposure to some substances may produce dermatitis if there is also exposure to sunlight (photodermatitis).

Certain occupational exposures may cause specific types of skin disease. For example, exposure to PCBs or dioxins may cause chloracne. Arsenic exposure may cause a specific type of skin lesion called arsenical dermatitis (arsenical warts).

Lung Disease

Although good surveillance data are not available on the incidence of chronic pulmonary diseases, they usually are regarded as a major type of occupational illness. The following are some important categories of occupational lung diseases (Parkes, 1982):

1. *Pneumoconiosis*. Exposure to some inorganic substances may cause a fibrogenic reaction in the lungs that leads eventually to a debilitating lung disease. The onset of illness is usually gradual, occurring many years after first exposure, although some cases may progress much more rapidly. These diseases can be detected by chest x-rays and by findings of restrictive disease on pulmonary function testing (if the disease is advanced). Examples of important pneumoconioses include asbestosis, silicosis, talcosis, coal workers' pneumoconiosis, and berylliosis.

2. *Byssinosis*. Chronic exposure to cotton dust may cause a pulmonary disease characterized by shortness of breath or wheezing when exposed to cotton dust, which eventually may lead to a condition similar to chronic bronchitis. The specific component of the cotton dust responsible for the disease is not known. Byssinosis is quite common among textile and other workers exposed to cotton dust and is known commonly as "brown lung."

3. *Chronic bronchitis*. Irritant dusts, fumes, or chemicals may cause a condition similar to chronic bronchitis. Symptoms may include productive cough, wheezing, shortness of breath, and frequent respiratory infections. Examples of occupational exposures that may cause bronchitis include welding fumes and sulfur dioxide.

4. *Asthma*. Certain organic chemicals and metals may produce allergic sensitization resulting in asthma. Typical symptoms include wheezing and shortness of breath, which sometimes do not occur until hours after leaving work; however, once a person is sensitized to the substance, even a slight exposure may trigger an asthmatic reaction. Examples of occupational exposures that may cause asthma include platinum, detergent enzymes, and isocyanates.

5. *Allergic alveolitis*. Exposure to some organic materials may cause a chronic lung disease due to pulmonary fibrosis. An immunological mechanism is responsible for the fibrosis. Typical symptoms include progressive shortness of breath and cough. Ex-

amples include mushroom workers' lung, coffee workers' lung, and farmers' lung.

Occupational Neurological Disease

Occupational exposure to many chemicals and metals may cause neurological damage (Spencer, 1980). Some of these substances act mainly on the central nervous system, while others primarily damage the peripheral nervous system. Peripheral neuropathy is usually characterized by gradual onset of muscle weakness and decreased sensation, generally starting in the hands and feet and spreading proximally. (These symptoms may vary depending on the toxic exposure.) After removal from exposure, affected persons usually recover, although they may not if the damage is severe. Occupational exposures causing peripheral neuropathy include lead, n-hexane, methyl butyl ketone, and organophosphate pesticides.

Some occupational exposures may cause damage to the central nervous system resulting in symptoms such as tremors (mercury) and psychological disturbance (lead, carbon disulfide, mercury). Chronic exposure to many solvents appears to cause some subtle damage to central nervous system functions (e.g., visual discrimination), which is detectable only by special psychological or behavioral tests.

Kidney Disease

Certain metals and chemicals may cause renal damage (NIOSH, 1977b). This toxicity is usually specific to certain parts of the kidney, resulting in specific functional disturbances. For example, cadmium and uranium exposure may result in renal tubular dysfunction, while chronic lead exposure may cause glomerular damage.

Liver Disease

Some occupational exposures cause liver damage (NIOSH, 1977b). In severe cases, there may be sufficient damage to cause jaundice and other biochemical signs of liver disease. Examples of occupational hepatotoxins include vinyl chloride, PCBs, and chloroprene. Infectious hepatitis is a major occupational disease for hospital workers, renal dialysis workers, and blood component manufacturing workers.

Heart Disease

Although a major cause of morbidity and mortality in the working population, the relationship between heart disease and occupational exposure is poorly understood. Some occupational exposures may exacerbate cardiovascular disease (carbon monoxide, carbon disulfide), while others may damage the cardiac muscle (cobalt).

Cancer

Estimates of the proportion of cancer deaths in the United States that may be caused by occupational exposures vary from 5 percent to 40 percent. This wide range of estimates is due mainly to the lack of sound surveillance data. There are many proven occupational carcinogens and many other occupational exposures suspected to cause cancer (Epstein, 1978; NIOSH, 1977a; Saffioti & Wagoner, 1976). A list of known occupational carcinogens is given in Table 6–2.

Usually, occupational cancers become manifest many years after the workers' first exposures; this waiting time is known as the latency period. Unlike many other toxic exposures, any exposure to a carcinogen appears to lead to some risk of cancer (i.e., there is no threshold dose). However, the degree of risk usually increases with increasing exposures. Individual susceptibility to occupational carcinogens is poorly understood; however, other risk factors (e.g., smoking) definitely increase the risk from exposure to an occupational carcinogen affecting the same site.

A major effort in the study of occupational carcinogens has been to develop methods for detecting potential occupational carcinogens before they are introduced into industry, causing large numbers of workers to develop cancer. Animal testing, cytogenetic

Table 6-2 Occupational Carcinogens

Carcinogen	Cancer Site	Examples of Exposed Occupations
1. 4-Aminodiphenyl Auramine B-napthylamine Magenta Benzidine	Bladder	Dye manufacturing; rubber manufacturing
2. Arsenic	Skin; lung; liver	Metal smelting; arsenic pesticide production; metal alloy workers
3. Asbestos	Lung; mesothelium; gastrointestinal tract	Asbestos miners; insulators; shipyard workers
4. Benzene	Leukemia (blood-forming organs)	Petrochemical workers; chemists
5. Bischloromethyl ether (BCME)	Lung	Organic chemical synthesizers
6. Cadmium	Prostate	Cadmium alloy workers; welders
7. Chromium/Chromates	Lung; nasal sinuses	Chromate producers; metal workers
8. Coke oven emissions	Lung; kidney	Coke oven workers
9. Foundry emissions	Lung	Foundry workers
10. Leather dust	Nasal cavity; nasal sinuses; bladder	Shoe manufacturing
11. Nickel	Lung; nasal passages	Nickel smelting; metal workers
12. Radiation (x-rays)	Leukemia (blood-forming organs; skin; breast; thyroid; bone)	Radiologists; industrial radiographers; atomic energy workers
13. Radon gas	Lung	Uranium and feldspar miners
14. Soots, tars, and oil (aromatic hydrocarbons).	Skin; lung; bladder; scrotum	Roofers; chimney sweepers; petroleum workers; shale oil workers
15. Ultraviolet light	Skin	Outdoor workers
16. Vinyl chloride	Liver; brain; lung	Polyvinyl chloride synthesizers; rubber workers
17. Welding fumes	Lung	Welders
18. Wood dust	Nasal passages	Hardwood workers; furniture makers

studies, and mutagenicity testing (e.g., Ames test) are major types of testing developed for early identification of potential human carcinogens. Although the extrapolation of the results of these laboratory tests to human occupational or environmental exposures is difficult (particularly the dose–response relationship), this type of testing has provided a very useful tool in the prevention of the occurrence of occupational cancer.

Another major public health problem is the past exposure of millions of workers to what now are known belatedly to be carcinogenic substances. For example, hundreds of thousands of workers were exposed to asbestos in shipyards in World War II.

Reproductive Hazards

The study of occupational reproductive hazards is a relatively new area of occupational health research, even though such effects have been suspected for many years (e.g., exposure to lead). As with occupational cancer, animal testing is an important mechanism for screening chemicals for reproductive toxicity and for understanding the pathophysiology of the effects better.

Several types of reproductive hazards are known (Thomas, 1981). Male infertility (lowered sperm counts) may be caused by exposure to lead, DBCP, Kepone, and a few other chemicals. Teratogenic agents may cause birth defects, miscarriages, low birth weight, and poor neurological development. Anesthetic gases, mercury, lead, and PCBs are examples of substances that may cause these health effects in exposed pregnant women. Many occupational exposures may cause genetic damage to the fetus. The sequelae of this may include miscarriages or birth defects. Tracing the effects of such exposures to reproductive outcomes is difficult, due to the many other factors affecting fetal development. Much of the current research in the area is focused on the development of approaches for evaluating reproductive toxicity.

Due to our poor understanding of reproductive effects and their sex specificity, policies for controlling exposure by restricting the exposure of one sex are complicated by the need to protect workers from job discrimination.

CONCLUSION

Due to the high incidence of occupationally related morbidity and mortality and the preventability of these outcomes, and because of increasing public awareness, occupational health will continue to be a growing area of public health concern. Considerable research must be conducted to help provide the information necessary for preventing occupationally related illness and death. Improved approaches to regulation and enforcement also are needed, so that research may be translated into preventive actions in the workplace.

REFERENCES

Armstrong T, Chaffin D (1979). Carpal tunnel syndrome and selected personal attributes. *J Occ Med 21*:481.

Billmaier D, Allen N, Craft B, et al. (1974). Peripheral neuropathy in a coats and fabrics plant. *J Occ Med 16*:665–671.

Bureau of Labor Statistics (1980). *Occupational Injuries and Illnesses in the United States by Industry, 1978.* Washington, D.C.: U.S. Government Printing Office.

California Department of Industrial Relations (1982). *Occupational Skin Disease in California, 1977.* Sacramento, Calif.

Cannon SB, Veazey JM, Jr., Jackson RS, Burse VW, Hayes C, Straub WE, Landrigan PJ, Liddle JA (1978). Epidemic Kepone poisoning in chemical workers. *Am J Epidemiol 107*:529–537.

Chaffin D (1975). Biochemics of manual materials handling and low-back pain. In Carl Zenz (ed), *Occupational Medicine Principles and Practical Applications.* Chicago: Year Book Medical Publications.

Chambers EG, Yule GU (1941). Theory and observation in the investigation of accident causation. *J Stat Soc 7*:89–109.

Epstein S (1978). The politics of cancer. San Francisco: Sierra Club Books.

Falk H, Creech JL, Jr., Heath CW, et al. (1974). Hepatic disease among workers at a vinyl chloride polymerization plant. *JAMA 230*:59.

Haddon W, Jr., Suchman EA, Klein D (1964). *Accident Research: Methods and Approaches.* New York: Harper & Row.

Herskowitz A, Ishii N, Schaumburg H (1971). n-Hexane neuropathy. *N Engl J Med 285*:82–85.

House Committee on Labor (1936). An investigation relating to health conditions of workers employed in the construction and maintenance of public utilities. Hearings before Special Subcommittee, January and February. Washington, D.C.: U.S. Government Printing Office.

Hueper WC (1942). *Occupational Tumors and Allied Diseases.* Springfield, Ill.: Charles C Thomas.

Kimbrough RD (ed) (1980). *Halogenated Biphenyls, Terphenyls, Napthalenes, Dibenzodioxins, and Related Products.* New York: Elsevier.

Kreiss K, Wegman DH, Niles CA, Siroky MB, Krane RJ, Feldman RG (1980). Neurological dysfunction of the bladder in workers exposed to dimethylaminoproprionitrile. *JAMA 243*:741-745.

Lainhart-Morgan WKC (1971). Extent of distribution of respiratory effects in coal miners. In MN Key (ed) *Pulmonary Reaction to Coal Dust.* New York: Academic Press.

Landrigan P (1981). Arsenic — State of the art. *Am J Ind Med 2*:5-14.

Lee J, White K (1980). A review of the health effects of cadmium. *Am J Ind Med 1*:307-317.

Lemen R, Johnson WM, Wagoner JK, et al. (1976). Cytological observations and cancer incidence following exposure to BCME. *Ann NY Acad Sci 271*:71-80.

Lemen R, Dement J (eds) (1979). *Dusts and Diseases.* Park Forest, Ill.: Pathotox Publishers.

Lloyd W (1975). Angiosarcoma of the liver in vinyl chloride/polyvinyl chloride workers. *J Occ Med 17*:333.

National Institute for Occupational Safety and Health (1977a). Chemical Carcinogens. In *Occupational Diseases: A Guide to Their Recognition.* Cincinnati, Ohio: National Institute for Occupational Safety and Health, DHEW (NIOSH) publication no. 77-181.

National Institute for Occupational Safety and Health (1977b). Chemical Hazards. In *Occupational Diseases: A Guide to Their Recognition.* Cincinnati, Ohio: National Institute for Occupational Safety and Health, DHEW (NIOSH) publication no. 77-181.

National Institute for Occupational Safety and Health (1977c). Dermatoses. In *Occupational Diseases: A Guide to Their Recognition.* Cincinnati, Ohio: National Institute for Occupational Safety and Health, DHEW (NIOSH) publication no. 77-181.

National Institute for Occupational Safety and Health (1977d). *National Occupational Hazard Survey: Survey Analysis and Supplemental Tables.* Cincinnati, Ohio: National Institute for Occupational Safety and Health, DHEW (NIOSH) publication no. 78-114.

National Institute for Occupational Safety and Health (1977e). *Occupational Exposure to Waste Anesthetic Gases and Vapors.* Cincinnati, Ohio: National Institute for Occupational Safety and Health, DHEW (NIOSH) publication no. 77-11250.

National Institute for Occupational Safety and Health (1977f). Oscillatory vibrators. In *Occupational Diseases: A Guide to Their Recognition.* Cincinnati, Ohio: National Institute for Occupational Safety and Health, DHEW (NIOSH) publication no. 77-181.

National Institute for Occupational Safety and Health (1977g). Pesticides. In

Occupational Diseases: A Guide to Their Recognition. Cinc\
National Institute for Occupational Safety and Health, DHE\
publication no. 77-181.

National Institute for Occupational Safety and Health (1977h). Radi.
Occupational Diseases: A Guide to Their Recognition. Cincinnati, Ol.
tional Institute for Occupational Safety and Health, DHEW (NIOSH,
lication no. 77-181.

National Institute for Occupational Safety and Health (1978). *Reducing Psycho-logical Stress.* Cincinnati, Ohio: National Institute for Occupational Safety and Health, DHEW (NIOSH) publication no. 78-140.

National Institute for Occupational Safety and Health (1981a). *Vibration White Finger Diseases in U.S. Workers Using Pneumatic Chipping and Grinding Handtools.* Cincinnati, Ohio: National Institute for Occupational Safety and Health, DHHS (NIOSH) publication no. 81-101.

National Institute for Occupational Safety and Health (1981b). *Work Practices Guide for Manual Lifting.* Cincinnati, Ohio: National Institute for Occupational Safety and Health, DHHS (NIOSH) publication no. 81-122.

National Institute for Occupational Safety and Health (1982). *Biological Effects of Infrared Radiation.* Cincinnati, Ohio: National Institute for Occupational Safety and Health, DHHS (NIOSH) publication no. 82-109.

National Institute of Health (1978). *Estimates of the Fraction of Cancer in the United States Related to Occupational Diseases.* Bethesda, Md.: U.S. Department of Health, Education and Welfare.

Nothstein G (1981). *The Law of Occupational Safety and Health.* New York: The Free Press.

Parkes WR (1982). *Occupational Lung Disorders*, 2nd ed. London: Butterworth & Company.

President's Report on Occupational Safety and Health (1972). Washington, D.C.: U.S. Government Printing Office.

Rehn L (1875). Blasonwulste bei fuschin-arbeitern. *Arch Klin Chir 50*:588–600.

Saari J, Lahtela J (1981). Work conditions and accidents in three industries. *Scand J Work Env Health 74*:97–105.

Saffioti U, Wagoner JK (1976). Occupational carcinogenesis. *Ann NY Acad Sci 271*:516.

Spencer P (1980). *Experimental and Clinical Neurotoxicology.* Baltimore: Williams and Wilkins.

Tanaka S (1975). Manganese. In Carl Zenz (ed), *Occupational Medicine Principles and Practical Applications.* Chicago: Year Book Medical Publications.

Thomas J (1981). Reproductive hazards and environmental chemicals: A review. *Toxic Substances Journal 2*:318–348.

United States Department of Labor (1980). *Interim Report to Congress on Occupational Diseases.* Washington, D.C.: U.S. Department of Labor.

Wasserman DE, Badger DW, Doyle TE, Margolies L (1974). Occupational vibration—An overview. *Am Soc Saf Eng J 19*:19–38.

Whorton D, Milby TH, Krauss RM, Stubbs, HA (1979). Testicular function in DBCP-exposed pesticides workers. *J Occ Med 21*:161–166.

Whorton MD, Milby TH (1980). Recovery of testicular function among DBCP workers. *J Occ Med 22*:177–179.

Appendix to Chapter 6: The Occupational Safety and Health Act

*Larry Auerbach**

Unlike other laws regulating environmental hazards, the Occupational Safety and Health Act of 1970 (OSHA) does not regulate the environment at large or purport to provide protection for the public at large. This act is designed to eliminate hazards in the specific limited environment of the workplace and to protect employees in that environment.

OSHA applies to all businesses affecting interstate commerce. The term "affecting interstate commerce" has been construed so broadly that substantially all employers are covered by this act. OSHA requires that each employer

1. Shall furnish to each of his employees employment and a place of employment which are free from recognized hazards that are causing or likely to cause death or serious physical harm to his employees

---

*This appendix was written by Larry Auerbach in his private capacity. No official support or endorsement by the U.S. Environmental Protection Agency or any other agency of the federal government is intended or should be inferred.

2. Shall comply with the occupational safety and health standards promulgated pursuant to (OSHA) [29USC §654(a)(1)]

The first section of this mandate is known as the "general duty clause." It makes it the duty of employers to free their workplaces of certain types of hazards, even though no specific federal regulation addresses the hazard. The hazards addressed under this clause must be both "recognized" and capable of causing death or serious physical harm. An employer will be found to have violated the general duty clause only if the hazard involved meets both tests.

A "recognized" hazard is one that is known to be hazardous by either the industry involved, safety experts knowledgeable of the industry, or by the particular employer. For example, if a condition has caused previous injury to employees, the employer obviously would know that it is a hazard. This condition therefore would be considered a "recognized" hazard. Also, if an industry organization such as the American National Standards Institute establishes safety procedures, it would be a "recognized" hazard for an employer to fail to follow those procedures.

A hazard is considered to be likely to cause death or serious physical harm based on what would happen if the injury that could occur did occur — not on the likelihood that it will occur. For example, a substance that causes minor skin rashes in 80 percent of exposed individuals would not fall into this category. A hazard that would result once in ten thousand cases in an employee losing an arm would fall into this category.

The second section of this mandate is the one that encompasses the great majority of issues under OSHA. That requirement is that employers comply with safety and health standards, that is, government regulations detailing specific safety and health requirements. These standards are printed in the Code of Federal Regulations and describe detailed safety requirements for a myriad of circumstances.

We will not discuss here the vast bulk of these regulations, which fall under the general classification of "safety" (fall protection, guarding of moving machinery parts, crane operation procedures, etc.). This discussion will be limited to "health" issues (carcinogens, toxic substances, etc.).

Federal regulations address a wide array of health issues. All such regulations are promulgated by the Secretary of Labor. While the Secretary of Labor has, in general, very broad discretion regarding establishing new regulations, OSHA provides specific guidance regarding exposure to what it terms "toxic materials or harmful physical agents." This term applies to carcinogens, lead, harmful chemicals, and so on.

OSHA requires that the standard set by the Secretary of Labor be that which protects an employee even if he/she is regularly exposed to the condition throughout his/her working life. The level of protection required is that which ensures, to the extent feasible, that no employee will have his/her health or ability to function materially impaired. There is a specific requirement that the Secretary of Labor, in setting such standards, rely on the latest available scientific data and evaluate the feasibility of the standards set.

Regulations promulgated under this act cover a myriad of potential health hazards. The requirements are often quite specific, based on the exact nature of the hazard and the measures believed necessary to protect employees.

A discussion of each health issue under OSHA would require literally volumes. For example, there are specific requirements regarding several carcinogens. These requirements detail standards for restricting access to areas of possible exposure, requiring protective clothing, ensuring proper ventilation, developing emergency plans, notifying employees of hazards, and so on.

MAXIMUM EXPOSURE LIMITS

OSHA regulations provide for maximum permissible exposure levels for literally hundreds of toxic substances. Specific regulations delineate safety requirements related to exposure to substances such as coal tar pitch volatiles, lead, asbestos, arsenic, and vinyl chloride. Certain OSHA regulations require different levels of compliance or time frames for achieving compliance in different operations or industries, depending on factors such as technological differences.

Maximum exposure limitations sometimes are expressed as "ceiling limits" — the maximum allowable concentration at any time in the workplace. Other limits are expressed in terms of the eight-hour time-weighted average (TWA). As an example, the eight-hour TWA for benzoyl peroxide is 5 mg/m³. An employee in an atmosphere of 8 mg/m³ for four hours, 4 mg/m³ for three hours, and then no exposure for one hour would have an average exposure during the eight-hour workday of 5.5 mg/m³ and would therefore be overexposed.

The standards specify that overexposure is to be remedied by engineering or administrative controls whenever feasible. Engineering controls generally would involve methods of preventing the hazardous substance from getting into the workplace atmosphere or removing it from this atmosphere. Administrative controls generally involve rotation of jobs between the exposed employees and other employees, thus limiting any one employee's exposure to the substance.

When engineering and administrative controls are not feasible, employers may resort to other protective measures. These measures could include respirators and impervious clothing, among others. The standards, however, are based upon the opinion that employees will be protected best by ensuring that they do not work in hazardous atmospheres. This approach is considered more likely to ensure employee safety than that of relying on employees to use the necessary protective equipment consistently and properly.

EXAMPLES OF REGULATED HAZARDS

This section will examine regulation of three specific environmental factors under this act: noise, benzene, and cotton dust. These three were selected as factors that provide insight into the broader operation of OSHA. They demonstrate the approach that has been taken by the government in regulating workplace environmental hazards and the interaction between law and medical science in this regulation.

The regulation of employee exposure to excess noise serves as an example of the traditional government approach to worker protection. The discussion regarding exposure to benzene provides an example of the interaction of medical and legal issues. The discussion regarding cotton dust demonstrates the legal resolution of the extension of issues addressed in benzene regulation.

Noise

Excessive noise is an environmental factor that is known to have several adverse effects on those exposed to it. Not the least of these effects, of course, is loss of hearing up to and including deafness.

The permissible employee exposure to noise is based on both the sound level and its duration; thus, an employee could be exposed to sound levels of 90 decibels for up to eight hours per day without exceeding the OSHA maximum, but the maximum exposure to sound levels of 110 decibels is only half an hour per day. The standard involved includes a table of the maximum duration for various levels of exposure, given in Table A6-1. The table is structured so that total employee exposure cannot exceed the equivalent of exposure to 90 decibels for eight hours in any day.

Just as with toxic chemical exposure, standards that establish federal regulation of noise place primary emphasis on reducing the employees' exposure to excessive noise. The secondary emphasis is on reducing the effect of the excessive noise if the exposure itself cannot be limited adequately.

Engineering controls might include sound-absorbing screens, mufflers on air outlets, sound-absorbing ceilings, and the like. For reduction of exposure to noise, administrative controls would include actions such as employee rotation to lessen exposure time or requir-

Table A6-1 Permissible Noise Exposures

Duration per Day (hr)	Sound Level dBA
8	90
6	92
4	95
3	97
2	100
1½	102
1	105
½	110
¼ or less	115

ing employees to leave a work area during portions of automatic processes.

If administrative and engineering controls cannot reduce employee noise exposure to permissible levels, they still are necessary if they will reduce the exposure substantially. In addition, if any overexposure remains, employers also must require employees to use personal protective devices, such as earplugs or earmuffs.

In deciding whether controls are feasible, both technological and economic aspects are considered; for example, an employer cannot use earplugs instead of engineering controls just because they are cheaper. The employer would have to demonstrate that significant reduction of the noise exposure would not be feasible otherwise. Only after such a demonstration could the employer rely on personal protective equipment in lieu of engineering or administrative controls.

Whenever employees are exposed to excess noise, the employer must implement a hearing conservation program. Such a program would include not only use of personal protective equipment but also periodic audiometric testing of employees. When employees suffer hearing loss, the employer must refer them to an otolaryngologist for examination.

Benzene

Benzene is a carcinogen that has been shown to have a causal relationship to leukemia. An extremely widely used industrial chemical, benzene is used in many manufacturing processes and as an additive in gasoline.

The OSHA regulations regarding benzene provide significant insight into the relationship between medical science and law in administering this act.

OSHA standards have been established to limit employee exposure to benzene in various ways. These include a time-weighted average limit, a ceiling limit, and a dermal-/eye-contact limit.

The standard sets a "ceiling" exposure for benzene in a different manner from other ceilings. This exposure level is in terms of both the maximum exposure allowed at any moment and the maximum over a brief period. The ceiling exposure level for benzene originally was set at 25 parts per million (ppm), averaged over a 10-minute exposure period, or 50 ppm peak exposure.

The maximum time-weighted average exposure to benzene was set at 10 ppm. This standard involved averaging an employee's exposure over an eight-hour workday in the manner discussed earlier.

At the urging of the National Institute of Occupational Safety and Health (NIOSH) a new OSHA standard was promulgated in 1977. This standard sought to lower the ceiling exposure level of benzene to 5 ppm over 15 minutes and the time-weighted average to 1 ppm.

The basis for the decision to establish the new regulation was the Secretary of Labor's position that no safe exposure level can be determined for a carcinogen. The maximum permissible level, therefore, would be the lowest level technologically obtainable.

Based on this same position, dermal or eye contact with liquid benzene was prohibited by the new standard. The only exception to this prohibition was exposure resulting from an isolated incident, that is, an accident or some other cause that is not likely to recur.

A lawsuit was filed by the American Petroleum Institute, seeking to block the government's implementation of these new and more stringent requirements. The United States Supreme Court eventually became the final arbiter of the medical/legal question of the appropriate maximum level of employee exposure to benzene (Industrial Union Department, AFL-CIO v. American Petroleum Institute, and Marshall v. American Petroleum Institute, 448 US 607, 100 S. ct. 2844, 1980).

The evidence showed that the government could not demonstrate definite risks associated with exposure to benzene at low levels such as the former 10 ppm exposure limit. It also was shown that no studies existed to show that there would be less cancer or other significant employee injury from exposure to 1 ppm than from exposure to 10 ppm.

As to the dermal contact rule, the court noted that OSHA had no evidence available regarding skin absorption of benzene. Old studies on this issue had been inconclusive, and no studies had been conducted using new and relatively simple procedures. The government instead relied on its theory that there was no safe exposure level to carcinogens.

The Supreme Court, in viewing these facts, rendered a deci-

sion that has had major impact regarding OSHA control of all carcinogens and even other toxic substances. The court said that OSHA
was intended by Congress to make workplaces safe but not necessarily completely risk free. The court decided that the government
had to justify such standards based on the best available scientific
evidence. This evidence must show the standard to be reasonably
necessary for and appropriate to removing a significant risk of harm.
The government had not done that in this case and was therefore
prohibited from enforcing its new time-weighted average or dermal-/
eye-contact standards.

Cotton Dust

Cotton dust is an air-borne substance comprised of particles
resulting from the preparation and manufacture of cotton products.
Inhalation of cotton dust may cause various respiratory effects
termed "byssinosis" and commonly called "brown lung disease." This
disease has long been recognized as a serious and potentially disabling condition.

The disease itself is known as a "continuum disease"; that is,
it may exist anywhere on a continuum from causing shortness of
breath and some loss of pulmonary function to being a chronic, irreversible, obstructive pulmonary disease with the potential of creating
strain on cardiovascular functions and contributing to death by heart
failure.

Originally, the OSHA standard regarding cotton dust required
a maximum permissible exposure level (PEL) of 1000 micrograms
of cotton dust per cubic meter of air (1000 $\mu g/m^3$). Based on studies
showing direct linear correlation between levels of exposure to cotton dust and the incidence level of byssinosis and based upon extensive public hearings, OSHA promulgated a new standard. The new
standard set PELs of 200 $\mu g/m^3$ for yarn manufacturing, 750 $\mu g/m^3$
for weaving and slashing operations, and 500 $\mu g/m^3$ for the rest of
the cotton industry. The differences in PELs were based primarily
on a determination of what levels were feasible in the various operations.

The government rejected both industry demands for higher
PELs and union demands for lower PELs. It found that higher PELs

would increase unnecessarily the incidence of byssinosis. While it was found that lower exposure levels would lessen the incidence of byssinosis, lower PELs were found to be technologically infeasible.

Industry groups filed a lawsuit to prohibit the enforcement of this standard. As with the benzene case, the United States Supreme Court again was called upon to decide an issue that would have widespread impact on government enforcement of health protection rules under OSHA. The court's decision was issued June 17, 1981 (American Textile Manufacturers Inst., et al. *v.* Donovan, 452 US 490, 101 S. ct. 2478, 1981).

In this case the government had extensive studies supporting its conclusion that adopting the new standard would lead to a significantly reduced incidence of byssinosis. The government therefore met the test it had failed under the benzene case and thus supported its action. A new and significant issue, however, was raised in opposition to this regulation: cost–benefit analysis.

The primary question for this case was whether the government was required to compare the cost of compliance with a new standard, to the benefits to be derived from the standard. The Supreme Court found that no such comparison was necessary, since Congress in enacting OSHA already had decided the relationship between costs and benefits.

The court held that Congress had determined that the benefit of employee health was always to prevail over concerns of costs, whenever it was technologically and economically feasible to provide the protection. The court thus held that if the industry has the economic resources and technological ability to comply with a regulation, the government need not compare the benefits of compliance with the cost of doing so. This ruling was based on the language in OSHA establishing the level of employee protection as that which ensures, to the extent feasible, no material impairment of health or functioning ability.

The ruling by the U.S. Supreme Court did not turn out to be the final chapter on the OSHA cotton-dust standard. Both the promulgation of this standard and the argument before the Supreme Court occurred during the administration of President Carter. (The Court's ruling was issued after President Reagan took office.) On February 9, 1982, the Reagan administration announced that the government would reconsider this standard.

Specifically, the Assistant Secretary of Labor for Occupational Safety and Health caused a "notice of proposed rulemaking" to be published in the Federal Register (47 Fed. Reg. 5906, 1982). This notice requested comment from all sources on a wide variety of questions related to this standard. Topics for comment included the possibility of narrowing the definition of the term "cotton dust" and the possibility of allowing alternate methods of compliance for small businesses.

At the time of this writing these questions remain open for comment and no firm proposals for change have been made.

CONCLUSION

The preceding discussion cannot be taken as providing definitive guidelines for understanding all health issues under OSHA; however, it can be useful as an example of the state of the law regarding health questions in the workplace environment at the time of this writing. As with all relatively new legal matters, the state of the law in OSHA is in a constant state of flux. The trend of this change can be understood best by examination of judicial developments. Court rulings, decisions by the Secretary of Labor regarding emphasis or direction, and congressional modification can change this trend at any time.

Chapter 7

Hazardous Waste Management

John Lewis Carden, Jr.

The civilizations of the industrialized world have developed appetites for goods and energy in keeping with their massive capabilities for producing these commodities. The comfort, savings in labor, and entertainment provided by energy consumption and the color, practicality, and diversion provided by processed or synthetic goods are welcomed. Our civilization, however, is beginning to wake up to an aspect of these prizes that in the past it has chosen to neglect or at best treat in passing. The production of energy and processed or synthetic goods often generates byproducts as well, many of which are of no further use and some of which are hazardous to humans and the environment. Both the quantity and nature of the hazardous waste produced make its proper disposal imperative if we are to protect our own safety and health and leave a nurturing environment for our progeny.

DEFINITION

Just what is a hazardous waste? An operational definition of a hazardous waste is any material that is of no further use and cannot be disposed of safely by allowing it to enter the environment in its original form in an uncontrolled manner.

Properties of wastes that make them potentially hazardous include flammability, acute or chronic toxicity, radioactivity, the presence of pathogens, pyrophoricity, explosivity, or a tendency to react rapidly with other materials present, producing flammable or toxic gases or excessive heat. The actual health and environmental hazards created by wastes with such properties depend on additional factors, including the proximity of the waste to human populations, the effectiveness of environmental transport mechanisms, the rate of degradation of the waste, and bioamplification in the food chain.

GENERAL MANAGEMENT STRATEGIES

Effective hazardous waste management, then, can be based on one of four strategies: (1) modification of the dangerous properties of the waste so that the waste can be allowed to enter the environment safely, (2) storage of the waste in a facility that prevents its introduction into the environment, (3) recycling, and (4) eliminating its production. The first option generally is referred to as treatment, and techniques such as incineration, detoxification, neutralization, reaction, solidification, encapsulation, and biological degradation may be used. For some wastes, especially those containing hazardous components that occur naturally in the environment, dilution of the waste with subsequent dispersal may be an acceptable treatment technique. Some wastes are produced for which technologies capable of converting them into environmentally acceptable form are not yet available. These wastes require secure, long-term storage. In some cases these wastes also are modified before storage to reduce the space occupied or to improve their storage stability. While these modifications do not make the waste environmentally acceptable, they also are often referred to as treatment. In this chapter, however, *treatment* will be used to denote a waste modification that eliminates the need for secure storage. Successful management of hazardous waste by storage requires well-designed facilities, routine monitoring, and long-term maintenance.

The proper disposal of hazardous waste is frequently costly; thus, as the management of hazardous waste has improved, the associated costs have made the recycling of some wastes economically attractive. As costs continue to increase in the future, the number of waste types that can be recycled may well increase, not only lessening environmental hazards but also providing better resource management. "Waste exchanges" are being organized around the United States to take advantage of this new market.

A long-term approach to hazardous waste management is to eliminate its production. This objective can be achieved in two ways: development of processes that do not produce any waste or the grouping of industries so that the complex as a whole converts all raw materials into products with no residual waste. The Soviet Union has adopted this so-called "low-waste" or "no-waste" approach for the management of its industrial chemical wastes (Zaytsev, 1982).

TYPES OF WASTES

Hazardous wastes can be divided into three broad categories: radioactive, infective, and chemical. Management of infective wastes virtually always involves treatment, while control of radioactive waste often utilizes secure storage. Management of chemical wastes is a complex combination of treatment and storage. The remainder of this chapter deals with problems and management techniques associated with each category of waste.

MANAGEMENT OF RADIOACTIVE WASTE

The first substantial quantities of radioactive wastes were generated in the early 1940s during the Manhattan Project. Fortunately, the hazards associated with these wastes were recognized early, and, in general, care was taken to prevent their widespread distribution in the environment.

Radioactive wastes normally are subdivided into two categories: high-level and low-level wastes. The distinction between these two types is not sharp, but the management techniques associated with them are quite different. Low-level waste normally is taken to mean a radioactive waste containing less than 10 nanocuries per gram of long-lived alpha-emitting isotopes. Furthermore, low-level wastes generally have sufficiently low beta-gamma activity to make cooling unnecessary, and they produce levels of penetrating radiation that do not require substantial shielding or remote manipulation for safe handling. Radioactive wastes that do not have those characteristics are considered high-level.

The practical task of assigning a particular waste to one group or the other usually is straightforward. High-level wastes are composed of items such as spent fuel elements from reactors; transuranic wastes from reprocessing operations; and discarded radioactive sources from medical, research, and industrial activities. These wastes are characterized by high specific activity, that is, high radioactive emission per unit mass. Low-level waste streams are composed of items such as scintillation detector fluids; contaminated laboratory and hospital supplies, including laboratory coats and bench mats; and animal carcasses containing radioactive tracers. These wastes are characterized by low specific activity. A few materials, such as ion exchange resins used for radio chemical separations or reactor water clean-up, may have intermediate specific activities, placing them in the gray area between the two classes.

In the United States, radioactive waste generated in the private sector is referred to as commercial waste, while that generated at government installations is referred to as defense waste. High- and low-level wastes are produced in both sectors. Disposal of commercial waste is regulated by the Nuclear Regulatory Commission, while defense waste disposal is regulated by the Department of Energy. Commercial and defense wastes are disposed of at different facilities, with the exception of the disposal of some high-level commercial waste at defense facilities.

High-level Radioactive Waste

Some characteristics of high-level wastes severely complicate adequate management. These characteristics include high radiation fields, large amounts of isotopes with long half-lives; and heat generation.

Management of these wastes has two essential components: (1) insuring that the waste is in a form (packaging system) that will not dissolve or otherwise allow natural transport mechanisms (groundwater movement, etc.) to carry the radioisotopes into the open environment; (2) providing adequate shielding and barriers (a repository) reliable over very long periods of time (Eichholz, 1976).

Currently, no commercial facility is available in the United

States for providing terminal storage of high-level wastes. The ongoing National Waste Terminal Storage Program (NWTS), established in 1976 by what then was called the U.S. Energy Research and Development Administration, has the goal of providing at least one fully operational repository for high-level waste before the turn of the century. The design requirement for this facility is that it be capable of preventing the escape of *any* of the stored radioactive waste into the biosphere for at least 1000 years. Meeting this requirement necessitates the development of a packaging system for the wastes that will deteriorate very slowly and the identification of appropriate geological formations and repository designs for containing the waste. The packaging system must contain the waste and minimize leaching of radionuclides into ground water, which it is postulated will eventually infiltrate the repository.

The currently favored packaging system consists of fusion of the waste into a borosilicate glass matrix to produce a low-solubility waste form and storage of this glass in a canister with a titanium alloy jacket. It is anticipated that some wastes will contain a sufficiently high level of radioactivity to raise the temperature of the waste container system to approximately 500°C, dramatically increasing the difficulty in maintaining the stability required. Most proposed designs for high-level waste repositories involve the cutting of a deep subterranean network of horizontal tunnels with cylindrical shafts cut into the tunnel floors to accept the waste canisters. A geological formation adequate for housing such a repository must provide, at minimum, protection from earthquakes and not fracture excessively as a result of the high temperatures produced by the waste. High ion-exchange capacity in the material surrounding the waste containers is also desirable, to inhibit the transport of radionuclides should the container system be breached. Basalt formations and salt domes are the prime candidates for geological repository media, with granite and tuff formations also under study (Battelle Memorial Institute, 1981).

Low-level Radioactive Waste

The management of low-level waste also utilizes storage, but the degree of isolation and longevity demanded of the storage facility is much reduced. Shallow land burial sites have been in operation for decades, including a number of privately owned and operated facilities. The number of commercial sites has dwindled, however, until only three remain in operation in the United States. They include facilities at Barnwell, South Carolina; Richland, Washington; and Beatty, Nevada. The total combined capacity of these sites is approximately 2.6 million cubic meters, while the projected annual rate of low-level waste production by 1990 is 0.18 million cubic meters.

To meet future needs for storage capacity and to provide for disposal near the site of production, the Low-Level Radioactive Waste Policy Act (PL 96-573) was enacted in December 1980. The act stipulates that, after January 1, 1986, states, or groups of states forming compacts, that have operational low-level waste disposal facilities can restrict access to these facilities to waste generators within the boundaries of the state or compact. Shortly after passage of the act, the Department of Energy (DOE) formed the Low-Level Waste Management Program to provide assistance to states or compacts in assuring the availability of operational facilities in all regions of the United States by the 1986 deadline (Large, 1981). The Nuclear Regulatory Commission (NRC) is currently formulating regulations for the management of low-level waste.

The overriding objective of low-level radioactive waste management is the protection of the health and safety of the public (Watson, 1979). Achieving this objective requires careful consideration of all aspects of the management program, including transportation, waste form, facility design, maintenance, and monitoring.

Transportation.   Transportation of any hazardous material poses risks because of reduced control. Any one of a number of possible — albeit improbable — events during transport could lead to an uncontrolled release of the waste into the environment. The transportation of radioactive waste is highly regulated to minimize risk. Low-level waste must be packed in strong, tight containers, to minimize the possibility for release into the environment in case of an accident. In addition, all liquid waste must be solidified, to slow dispersion through the environment if the container is breached. The regulations for transportation and packaging of low-level waste are promulgated by the Department of Transportation. Safe and effective response to a transportation accident requires detailed knowledge of the contents; thus manifests are required under both the DOT regulations and the proposed NRC regulations.

Forms of Waste.   Low-level waste is generated in an extremely diverse array of forms, including aqueous solutions, contaminated organic solvents, paper, animal carcasses, wood, and cinder blocks. The form of the waste impacts strongly on disposal. Bulky wastes with low specific activity take up a disproportionate share of the volume available in the disposal facility. Since this space has a very high intrinsic value, volume reduction techniques are used on such wastes whenever feasible, leaving a residue with much higher specific activity. Compaction, evaporation, and incineration are the most common volume-reduction techniques. Appropriate measures must be taken to prevent radionuclides or other hazardous materials from entering the environment as a result of these procedures.

A number of materials are being investigated to identify matrices into which waste can be incorporated to render the radionuclides resistant to leaching by ground water infiltrate. These materials include asphalt cement, plastics, and glasses. While the long-term stability of waste in these materials is still under investigation, many are currently used commercially to improve waste retention in landfills.

Waste form also has an effect on the stability of the filled and sealed burial trench. In some of the early burial grounds, such as those at Oak Ridge, Tennessee, biodegradable materials were loaded into the trenches. As degradation of these materials occurred, the accompanying volume reduction led to subsidence and failure of the trench caps (Webster, 1979). Large holes actually appeared in some. This resulted in rapid infiltration with subsequent contamination of surface water. Biodegradation of organic wastes also has been observed to increase the acidity of water in the trench, making it more effective in dissolving the radionuclides present in the waste, thus leading to a more concentrated leachate.

Methane gas is formed as a result of the anaerobic bacterial activity in some waste materials. This can lead to the formation of gas pockets and also can provide a carrier gas that increases the rate of vapor transport of gaseous radionuclides into the atmosphere.

A high-density, nonleachable, and nonbiodegradable solid would be an ideal waste form. Tritium-containing liquids cannot be concentrated or solidified readily; thus, they pose a special problem.

Facility Design.   Since disposal of most low-level waste currently involves near-the-surface land burial, the ability of water infiltrate to leach radionuclides from waste matrices is an important consideration. Once suspended or in solution, a number of mechanisms may result in transport into and throughout the environment. Radionuclides can leave a burial trench by percolation through its sides or bottom or, if the trench becomes saturated, by overflow into surface water. Once waste has traversed the trench sides or bottom, it can migrate into water-bearing strata and contaminate the local aquifer. Soils with high ion exchange capacity tend to bind strongly with many ionic radionuclides, thus retarding their migration until the ion exchange capacity of the soil is exceeded. Once saturated, the soil provides no further retardation. Soil with low permeability also retards migration, and since permeability, unlike ion exchange, is not limited by capacity, it represents a permanent barrier, provided channels do not develop. If, on the other hand, the trench fills with water and overflows, causing surface water to become contaminated, the waste may move rapidly through the environment.

At this time, all of the methods being considered seriously for the ultimate disposal of low-level radioactive waste involve land burial. Two types of approaches are being considered: shallow land burial and so-called greater confinement techniques. Shallow land burial has been the prevalent technique to this point. The identification of an appropriate geological formation for the siting of such a facility is critically important. Requirements include a mean water table well below the bottom of the trenches, uniformly impermeable soil to prevent percolation of leachate or other liquids from the cell, and trench elevation well above the flood plain to preclude massive washout. In areas that do not meet the water table and permeability criteria, engineered trenches or cells that present human-made barriers to migration into or from the cell have been proposed. This approach will be discussed in more detail under chemical waste disposal.

The greater confinement options currently under consideration essentially provide for burial at a greater depth with a thicker trench cap. Shallow land burial normally involves trenches less than 10 meters deep, while greater confinement plans normally call for trenches of from 15 to 30 meters deep, with proportionately thicker caps.

The success of shallow land burial depends largely on preventing water infiltration and saturation of the burial trench. Infiltration can occur through any of the trench boundaries. Serious problems have been encountered in providing long-term cap integrity at humid sites, such as the former burial ground at Maxey Flats in Kentucky (Legislative Research Commission, 1980). Caps normally are made by building up layers of compacted clay over the cell to a depth of from one to three meters. Waste subsidence, thermal cycling, and intrusion by roots and small animals have led to frequent cap failures (Meyer, 1976). Water infiltration through permeable trench sides, as occurred in West Valley, New York (Meyer, Giardina, DeBonis, & Eng, 1977), also has led to the introduction of radionuclides into the environment. Improved trench and cap design as well as better control over waste form are needed to reduce the incidence of failure in trench confinement.

Maintenance and Monitoring.   Long-term maintenance and monitoring are essential for ensuring confinement in a waste burial site. Current plans under the Low-Level Waste Management Program are for provision of active site maintenance for 100 years after the site has stopped receiving waste and a closure plan has been executed. The objective of the closure plan is to stabilize the site so that natural processes will not lead to the release of radionuclides (Murphy & Holter, 1980). The plan normally includes contouring the earth over the trenches to minimize erosion, providing sufficient topsoil to ensure the growth of a plant cover, and the construction of fences or other barriers to prevent intrusion by unauthorized persons. Permanent markers or monuments also would be constructed, to provide warning of potential hazards below the surface.

The Low-Level Waste Management Program anticipates that activity during the 100-year maintenance phase will be restricted to monitoring, grass mowing, and fence mending. A study of maintenance requirements following closure (Johnson, Warren, & Lynch, 1977), prompted by the water intrusion problems experienced at Maxey Flats, concluded that recapping of trenches also was likely to be required if the trenches were to remain free of water. The problems associated with long-term prevention of migration of radionuclides from well-planned and executed burial sites probably will depend on climatic conditions more than any other factor, with sites in humid regions presenting the most difficult problems. If only solidified wastes are deposited into these sites, waste migration is much less likely to become a problem.

MANAGEMENT OF INFECTIOUS WASTE

The distinguishing characteristic of infectious waste is the presence of pathogenic organisms. Such wastes are produced by medical and veterinary facilities, research laboratories, and some manufacturing operations that make use of biological processes. While federal regulation of the disposal of radioactive waste is highly developed, quite the opposite is true for infectious waste. Under the authority granted in Section 4005(c) of the Resource Conservation and Recovery Act of 1976 (RCRA), the Environmental Protection Agency prohibits the open dumping of infectious wastes unless measures have been taken to minimize disease vectors. Many states have a more developed regulatory structure for the disposal of these wastes, and indeed the EPA is in the process of promulgating comprehensive regulations under RCRA.

Infectious wastes differ from radioactive and chemical wastes in that it is often possible through decontamination to reduce the hazard to a level that allows disposal by ordinary means. The success of a decontamination technique depends on the pathogen present and the nature of the contaminated material. Decontamination agents generally fall into one of four categories: heat, liquid chemicals, gases and vapors, and radiation.

Heating with pressurized steam at 121° C (autoclaving) generally is considered the most convenient and effective method of sterilization. Dry heating, even at substantially higher temperatures, can be less effective if the material being decontaminated does not have rapid and uniform heat transfer characteristics.

Liquid chemicals often are used to decontaminate surfaces and bulk liquid wastes. The effectiveness of these decontaminants is dependent on a number of factors, including temperature; contact time; pH; the relative concentrations of the decontaminant; the pathogen and interfering substances present; the degree of contact between the decontaminant and pathogen, which depends on mixing, formation of emulsions on colloids, and so forth; and the toxicity of the decontaminant to the pathogen. Common liquid decontaminants include ethyl and isopropyl alcohol, formaldehyde, phenol, quarternary ammonium compounds, chlorine, and iodine. A potential problem in the use of chemical decontaminants is the conversion of an infectious waste into a hazardous chemical waste.

Fumigant vapors and gases are used to decontaminate large structures, delicate instruments, or other items that cannot be heated or wetted. The most useful decontaminants of this type are formaldehyde and ethylene oxide. Unfortunately, both of these materials are believed to pose serious health risks to those using them. The National Institute for Occupational Safety and Health (1981) has recommended that, as a prudent public health measure, formaldehyde be considered an occupational carcinogen and that exposure be held to the lowest level feasible. Ethylene oxide is a genotoxin with safe exposure limits still being debated.

Ultraviolet radiation is highly bactericidal, with the maximum bactericidal action spectrum for *E. coli* occurring at 160 nanometers. However, the low penetrating power of ultraviolet radiation generally limits its applicability to surface decontamination. More penetrating radiations have been used for special applications, but precautions are required to protect personnel involved.

Infectious waste that has not been decontaminated or sterilized generally is disposed of by incineration. The design of the incineration system must take into account both the resistance of the pathogens present and regulations relating to air quality.

MANAGEMENT OF HAZARDOUS CHEMICAL WASTE

Until quite recently, the management of hazardous chemical waste was an activity of little interest to anyone other than those directly involved. Now it has become a political issue of unrivaled emotional strength, involving a very broad spectrum of individuals and groups in the United States.

The current U.S. capacity for the disposal of hazardous chemical waste in licensed facilities is inadequate, and the few existing facilities are remote from many of their customers. There has been an attempt in the last few years to open new disposal facilities, in order to increase licensed disposal capacity and provide for disposal nearer the site of waste generation. Some of these attempts have led to bitter controversy, the destruction of property, and death threats.

Few issues have focused so finely the conflict between the rights of individuals and the collective needs of our society. Some individuals oppose such facilities because of fears for their health and damage to their local environment. Government, on the other hand, strongly encourages the development of new facilities because without them adequate control of hazardous chemical waste disposal is virtually impossible. Hazardous chemical waste is generated with or without adequate disposal facilities and regulatory control, leading to practices like "midnight dumping." These practices represent a serious threat to the general population and the environment, exemplified by the dioxin contamination problem around Times Beach, Missouri, which was present for many years before it was recognized.

Protection of public health and the environment demands that the conflicts surrounding adequate chemical waste management be resolved. The technology base is developing rapidly, and these developments may hold the key to a risk–benefit formula that will satisfy all legitimate concerns.

Potential Environmental Pathways

Widely publicized failures in hazardous chemical waste management in the United States — Elizabeth, New Jersey and Love Canal in New York — represent only the "tip of the iceberg," with hundreds of additional cases on file with the EPA. The vast majority of these cases involve the open dumping of wastes into improperly operated landfills or surface impoundments. Dumping of liquid wastes into natural depressions or abandoned mine shafts, burial of liquid or solid wastes in trenches dug into permeable geological strata, abandoning 55-gallon drums of waste in open uncontrolled areas, mixing toxic liquids with fuel oil distributed to residential customers, and disposal of hazardous wastes in municipal sanitary landfills are all to be found among the dangerous and often criminal practices of the past. Numerous incidents have resulted in exposure of local populations to toxins, with illness resulting. The most common mode of transport of these materials through the environment to human populations has been via water, either surface or ground.

Surface Water. Surface water contamination has played a role in such famous incidents as the so-called "Valley of the Drums" in Bullitt County, Kentucky. In this incident, a multicolored oily mixture was discovered flowing into a creek from leaking drums at a

23-acre site containing more than 20,000 — and perhaps as many as 200,000 — 55-gallon drums. Remedial action included damming the creek and treating the contaminated water before its release. Cleanup of this site cost the public approximately $300,000 (Smith, 1980).

The public health hazard posed by surface water pollution depends on many factors, the most obvious being the ultimate use of the water. Incidents involving a rapid release, such as precipitation-induced washout of an impoundment, usually represent a limited health threat because of the lack of subtlety. An oily film, color, or unusual smell often warns that a stream has been polluted. The fact that the pollution source generally is located above ground where it is visible also often leads to recognition of the presence of a problem before serious human health effects are observed. The gradual leaching of toxic materials, however, can pose a serious hazard.

Groundwater.   Most incidents leading to illness have involved subsurface or groundwater pollution. The burial of a quantity of excess lead arsenate insecticide on the Perham, Minnesota fairgrounds in 1934 provides a classic example. In 1972, a construction company built a shop adjacent to the long-forgotten arsenic burial site and dug a well about 50 feet away from it. Shortly after the building was completed, 13 employees became ill. Approximately two weeks passed before the illness was diagnosed as arsenic poisoning, during which time other employees continued to drink the water. Two more workers became seriously ill, one requiring six months' convalescence.

Groundwater contamination is often insidious, and the source is sometimes very difficult to locate. Typically, hazardous waste is placed on the ground surface or is buried. If the waste is contained in steel drums, the drums corrode away within approximately six years unless the waste itself speeds up the process. Once the waste leaks out of its container, precipitation may begin to transport the waste through the soil toward the local aquifer. This transport may involve solubilization if the waste dissolves in water or emulsification or suspension if the waste is essentially insoluble but can be broken up into small stable droplets or particles. Most chemical wastes are mixtures; thus some components may dissolve while others form emulsions or suspensions, leaving behind the insoluble components.

Once in the aquifer, the waste continues to move, now directed toward a discharge point, which may be a spring, creek, or well. The rate of movement depends on the structure of the aquifer and its recharge rate. Under normal conditions, water movement of a few meters per day would be expected in sand, gravel, fractured limestone, or dolomite, while movement in sandstone, clay, or shale would not be expected to exceed a few meters per year.

The slow movement through a solid matrix, characteristic of groundwater flow, tends to minimize mixing; thus the hazardous wastes finding their way into an aquifer may form a concentrated band or plume. If a well or some other discharge point intercepts this plume, the contaminant will reenter the surface environment. If this contaminated discharge contributes to a drinking water supply, the consequences can be quite serious. Once contaminated, the slow rate of water migration in some aquifers leads to very long cleanup times.

Air.   Surface and groundwater are by far the most important pathways for transporting hazardous waste through the environment. Transport through the atmosphere is possible, however, if the waste is in the form of dust, vapor, or gas. In cases where exposure does occur via the atmosphere, the extent of the resulting health hazard is often unclear. At Love Canal, for instance, vapors of toxic materials were detected in surrounding homes. The concentrations observed were generally well below those considered hazardous in the industrial environment by the U.S. Occupational Safety and Health Administration. This does not necessarily imply that the exposures that occurred at Love Canal did not represent a hazard. OSHA exposure standards are written for an eight-hour time-weighted average exposure to pure compounds (see Chapter 6). Longer exposure times and exposure to mixtures, with the potential for synergistic effects, greatly complicate prediction of the hazard involved. OSHA standards also assume a working population, that is, a population that does not include the infirm, elderly, or the very young. Until it is possible to demonstrate scientifically a cause and effect relationship between air-borne exposure to toxic chemical wastes and adverse health effects, this route of exposure will continue to be of unknown significance in many cases.

Nevertheless, incidents have occurred that clearly demonstrate the potential for environmental damage from air-borne toxic chemicals. For example, in Seveso, Italy, in July 1976, a rupture disk on a 2,4,5-trichlorophenol reactor blew out, releasing a cloud containing three to 16 kilograms of a byproduct, 2,3,7,8-tetrachlorodibenzo-2,4-dioxin. Some residents quickly developed symptoms of dioxin poisoning, while the appearance of symptoms in others was delayed for a few days. Symptoms included erythema and skin burns, chloracne, abdominal pains, and internal bleeding. The documented potent teratogenic effect of this material in rats and mice produced great concern in the community and led to a number of induced abortions. A 200-acre area of the city was evacuated. Because of the persistence of 2,3,7,8-tetrachlorodibenzo-2,4-dioxin, 10 years or more may be required before natural processes can lower the dioxin concentration in the soil to a level that will allow safe habitation (Rawls & O'Sullivan, 1976).

Nature and Magnitude of the Problem

Public concern over the management of hazardous chemical waste in the United States was a major driving force behind the passage of two important bills designed to protect the environment and public health: (1) the Resource Conservation and Recovery Act of 1976 (RCRA) which regulates the management of hazardous waste currently being produced, and (2) the Comprehensive Environmental Response, Compensation and Liability Act of 1980 (Superfund), which provides funds and leadership for the cleaning up of abandoned hazardous waste sites. Both pieces of legislation are discussed later in this chapter and in Chapter 8. Epstein, Brown, and Pope (1982) have published an interesting history of the development of these bills.

One provision of RCRA, requirement of an annual report from all generators of hazardous wastes, was intended to provide a clear picture of hazardous waste production in the United States. Unfortunately, implementation and analysis of responses has been very slow, with the first preliminary data being released in September 1983. Prior to the release of these data, the EPA has estimated that approximately 40 million metric tons of hazardous waste were produced annually. The report indicated that total annual production in 1981 was in fact a staggering 150 million metric tons, with approximately 95 percent being managed on site. The remaining 5 percent was sent off site to licensed disposal facilities. Interestingly, 1 percent of the generators accounted for 90 percent of the hazardous waste produced. The highest waste production areas were found to be the Midwest and Middle Atlantic states.

Prior to the implementation of the RCRA regulations, the EPA (Kovalick, Corson, Day, et al., 1977), using the sketchy information available, made a projection of generation rates of key industries. The resulting information for the 10 largest producers is presented in Table 7-1. While the absolute accuracy of the data is questionable, they do give information about the relative importance of various categories of industries as waste generators. The amounts of waste generated are presented both in terms of the weight actually produced, "wet weight," and the weight of waste that would remain if the associated liquid were removed to the extent feasible.

The two categories generating the most waste — organic chemicals, pesticides, and explosives and primary metals — produce more than twice as much waste as the next two categories, electroplating and inorganic chemicals. However, in order to evaluate the contri-

Table 7-1   Amount of Hazardous Chemical Waste Generated in 1977 by the 10 Largest Producers

Industry	Hazardous Chemical Waste Production in 1977 (million metric tons)	
	Dry	Wet
1. Organic chemicals, pesticides, and explosives	3.5	11.7
2. Primary metals smelting and refining	4.7	9.1
3. Electroplating	1.3	4.1
4. Inorganic chemicals	2.3	3.9
5. Textile dying and finishing	0.50	1.9
6. Petroleum refining	0.72	1.8
7. Rubber and plastics	0.24	0.94
8. Batteries	0.08	0.16
9. Special machinery	0.09	0.15
10. Leather tanning	0.05	0.14

Source: W. W. Kovalick, Corson, Day, et al. *State Decision-Maker's Guide for Hazardous Waste Management*. Washington, D.C.: U.S. Environmental Protection Agency, EPA publication no. EPA SW-612.

Table 7-2 Percentage of Hazardous Waste Disposed of by Various Techniques, 1973–1975

Disposal Practice	Percent of Total Wet Weight of Potentially Hazardous Waste
Environmentally Inadequate	
Unlined surface impoundment	48.3
Nonsecure landfill (open dumps, etc.)	30.3
Uncontrolled incineration	9.7
Deep well injection	1.7
Land spreading	0.3
Use on roads	Less than 0.1
Sewered	Less than 0.1
TOTAL	90.4
Environmentally Adequate	
Controlled incineration	5.6
Secure landfill	2.3
Recovery	1.7
Lined surface impoundments	Less than 0.1
Waste-water treatment	Less than 0.1
Autoclaving	Less than 0.1
TOTAL	9.6

Source: W. W. Kovalick, Corson, Day, et al. *State Decision-Maker's Guide for Hazardous Waste Management*. Washington, D.C.: U.S. Environmental Protection Agency, EPA publication no. EPA SW-612.

bution of these industries to the nation's overall hazardous waste management problems, a number of other factors must be considered, including the hazards associated with the wastes produced and the ease with which the waste can be disposed of in an acceptable manner.

This same EPA report (Kovalick et al., 1977) also provided information on waste management practices between 1973 and 1975. Table 7-2 gives the most commonly reported disposal methods and the percentage of waste disposed of by each. These practices are divided into two categories: environmentally inadequate, that is, those practices posing a clear potential health and/or environmental hazard; and environmentally adequate, that is, those practices that should not pose a hazard. Note that only about 10 percent of the waste was disposed of using a method considered environmentally adequate.

In the past, adequate hazardous chemical waste management has been associated primarily with large companies possessing the financial and, perhaps more important, the technological resources required. Small manufacturers and nonmanufacturing generators, such as research facilities and hospitals, need access to competent and reliable assistance, because maintaining their own disposal capability is often prohibitively costly.

Hierarchy of Management Options

The evidence clearly indicates that for the most part, past management of hazardous chemical waste has been inadequate and must be modified in the future. Some waste management options are more desirable than others, and the EPA (Kovalick et al., 1977) has suggested the following hierarchy of options, starting with the most desirable:

1. Waste elimination or reduction at the source
2. Waste separation and concentration
3. Waste exchange
4. Energy and material recovery
5. Incineration or treatment
6. Secure land disposal

Some wastes require a combination of these options to provide the optimum waste management strategy. Presently the two most-used options for hazardous chemical waste management are secure chemical landfill storage and incineration. Thus, a more detailed discussion of these techniques will be included in the following discussion of all five options.

Waste Elimination or Reduction.   The ideal option is to eliminate or at least minimize hazardous waste production. This objective can be achieved to varying degrees by raw material substitution or process modification.

Waste Separation and Concentration.   If an irreducible amount of waste is being produced, the next option is to keep the various types of wastes segregated so that the most appropriate disposal technique can be used for each. It is also important to prevent these wastes from comingling with nonhazardous process waste streams, which would result in the generation of a large amount of dilute hazardous waste. There are some exceptions to this principle; for example, some acidic and basic waste streams can be combined, neutralizing both.

Waste Exchange. Properly concentrated and segregated wastes may represent a raw material for another process. The potential of this option is just beginning to be recognized, and waste exchanges and clearinghouses are beginning to appear all around the country.

Energy and Material Recovery. If a waste cannot be put to use in the form generated, it still may represent a valuable material or energy resource. In some cases wastes are the raw materials from which metals or synthetic chemicals can be recovered at a lower cost than through refining of naturally occurring minerals or through normal commercial synthetic processes. This type of recovery, however, has not been common practice in the past because it was often difficult to assure a sufficiently large and reliable supply of the waste to justify the capital outlay required. If the waste does not represent a cost-effective raw material for a useful product but has a reasonable heat content (stored chemical energy), energy recovery may be possible via combustion, which can be used to generate heat or electrical power. Air pollution abatement, however, is a serious concern.

Incineration or Treatment. If the waste does not represent a chemical or energy resource, then it should be destroyed by, for example, incineration or converted by treatment to a form that poses minimal risk if released into the environment. Technologies for the incineration of hazardous chemical wastes are developing rapidly, and a discussion of this option is presented later. *Treatment* is used here to denote waste modification techniques that reduce the hazard associated with a waste, thus allowing the treated waste to enter the environment without causing significant harm. Treatment techniques can be divided into one of three general categories: volume reduction, detoxification, and solidification or fixation.

1.   *Volume reduction.* Not all forms of volume reduction qualify as treatment techniques. Volume reduction by water removal or

concentration is sometimes referred to as treatment, but it does not meet the criteria because it rarely results in a more environmentally acceptable waste. Instead, concentration normally is practiced to conserve space in a chemical landfill. Incineration produces a large volume reduction. If a solid residue or clinker remains after incineration, it is often less hazardous than the original waste. Volume reduction by incineration, then, is a treatment technique.

2. *Detoxification.* This can involve any one of a number of processes. Spraying is used to remove volatile toxins from aqueous waste. Some toxic metals can be converted to highly insoluble and thus biologically inaccessible compounds; for instance, highly toxic soluble barium salts can be rendered virtually harmless by conversion to the sulfates. Cyanides can be destroyed by chlorine or other oxidizing agents. The carcinogenic Cr^{6+} ion can be reduced to a less hazardous oxidation state prior to disposal. Some biodegradable hazardous wastes can be detoxified by land farming, that is, mixing the waste into the topsoil in a secure area. This technique requires careful management to prevent off-site contamination and to maintain soil conditions within the productive range for the microorganisms involved. Other biodegradable wastes can be treated in surface impoundments.

3. *Solidification.* This involves converting waste into a solid form, usually by incorporation into a matrix. A good matrix material can incorporate diluted waste without significant changes in its physical strength or chemical stability. The purpose of solidification is to trap the waste in order to control the rate at which ground or surface water coming into contact with the waste can dissolve the hazardous components. With adequate control of release rates, the concentrations of hazardous components leaving the disposal site would be sufficiently low to pose no health or environmental hazard. In a few instances solidification involves polymerization of waste components, but more often it is achieved by mixing the waste with Portland cement or some proprietary agent to form an encapsulating matrix. In most cases, the long-term stability and leachability under landfill conditions of solidified wastes are unknown.

Controlled incineration is the most common form of environmentally adequate waste disposal. Incineration is a process in which heat and oxidation modify thermally labile materials. Combustible components are converted to oxides, usually accompanied by the release of additional heat. Some functional groups, such as covalently bonded chlorine, are reduced. Under appropriate conditions, unreactive components such as some inorganic salts are incorporated into a dense matrix with low solubility (a clinker). Incineration, then, converts hazardous waste components into less hazardous materials. Discounting the gaseous products, a very large reduction in volume also accompanies incineration.

Despite its advantages, incineration has seen rather limited use for hazardous waste disposal, largely because of cost. In 1978, it was estimated that incineration cost two to three times as much as burial in a chemical landfill (Sobel, 1978). As a result of the tighter regulations governing landfills and taxes being imposed upon them by state and local governments, the cost of these disposal options is now nearly equal.

Incineration is not without environmental hazards. Transportation of waste to an incinerator is, of course, no less risky than transportation to a landfill. Incineration has the potential for generating major air pollution problems; thus, systems have to be designed to provide adequate air pollution abatement and maintenance of comprehensive monitoring. If the off-gases are treated by water scrubbing, water pollution also can become a problem. Trial burns must be conducted on all new waste types to insure that the pollution control system is adequate. If a solid residue is produced, it must be characterized to determine if it is hazardous and, if so, treated accordingly.

A particularly useful form of incineration involves burning waste in a rotary kiln like those used to manufacture cement. The rotating drum provides good mixing and will even allow the disposal of some types of drummed waste, drum and all, thus eliminating unpacking at the disposal site.

The term *incineration* has been used, up to this point, in a generic sense. Incineration actually implies the burning of a material in at least a stoichiometric amount of oxygen, that is, enough oxygen to convert all of the carbon present to CO_2. Waste heated in the absence of oxygen, a process called *pyrolysis*, results in the conversion of the carbon present into oils or combustible solids and CO and other combustible gases. The oils, solids, and gases then may be used as heat sources. Another technique involves allowing less than a stoichiometric amount of oxygen into the heating zone. This process, usually called "starved air combustion," is more efficient than incineration and also leads to combustible products. A modification of this technique, called "slag-forming pyrolysis," utilizes a long reaction chimney with a high-temperature hearth at the bottom. The chimney is packed continually with municipal waste, including paper, plastics, cans, metal scrap, and so forth. Noncombustible hazardous waste can be mixed with the municipal waste. Pyrolysis occurs above the hearth and the waste disintegrates, moving down the chimney. The resulting pyrolysis gases are trapped and used to augment the fuel for pollution control afterburners. The temperature in the hearth is maintained at a level high enough to melt the solids in the waste, forming a slag and thus incorporating the hazardous wastes present into an insoluble matrix.

Another novel approach, called the MODAR process, utilizes a National Aeronautics and Space Administration (NASA) technology spinoff to destroy extremely stable materials efficiently. Examples include polychlorinated biphenyls, DDT, and wastes from the manufacture of explosives. The waste is injected into a stream of supercritical water ($T > 374°$ C, $P > 218$ atm.), where reforming (conversion to smaller molecules) occurs. Oxygen then is introduced, and the products of reforming are oxidized, raising the temperature to approximately 600° C. The reaction is essentially complete, and if the feed is at least five percent organic, enough energy can be recovered to make the system self-sustaining, that is, no additional energy need be provided. The complete oxidation of the waste greatly simplifies the air pollution control equipment required. The water recovered from the system is sufficiently pure that NASA is considering using this process for recycling water from metabolic waste on board future space stations.

Secure Land Disposal. The option at the bottom of the waste-management hierarchy is secure land disposal. Two somewhat different approaches to secure land disposal are practiced. One approach is similar to the operation of a sanitary landfill facility, where waste is placed in contact with soil to encourage biological degradation. A much higher degree of ground and surface water isolation is required, however, for chemical disposal. Unlike land farming, which involves mixing the waste into the surface of the soil, this approach may involve burial of bulk quantities of the waste under a thin covering of soil. A significant amount of biological treatment occurs in these facilities, and, if disposal is limited to biodegradable wastes, the residue may be environmentally acceptable. If such is the case, the ultimate closure of this type of facility would be no more difficult than a sanitary landfill. If nondegradable wastes are included, however, closure providing long-term protection could become very complicated and expensive. The Union Carbide Corporation and the Bayer Chemical Company of West Germany have operated such landfills for many years.

The other approach to secure land disposal is perpetual storage. Its objective is to isolate the waste from the environment by using some type of manufactured or natural barrier sufficiently stable to insure the prevention of an environmentally unacceptable release of hazardous waste at any point in the future. Design concepts that have been suggested to meet this objective will be discussed later.

Secure land disposal is placed last in the hierarchy of management options because of the uncertainty regarding long-term success and the potential need for human intervention from time to time to maintain the integrity of the site. Such intervention would add substantially to the cost of "disposal" by this option. These long-term costs need careful attention; otherwise, future generations will pay for our poor judgment and planning and in effect subsidize our lifestyle and prosperity. There is, however, a proper role for secure land disposal. The treatment of hazardous waste often results in a material that should not be allowed to enter the environment en masse but might be allowed to reenter safely via the slow process of reassimilation within an appropriately designed secure chemical landfill.

The majority of secure chemical landfill facilities currently operating or in the licensing process are of the perpetual storage type. As we have said, such facilities are intended to isolate the stored wastes from the environment until the wastes can be reassimilated safely. This period may be extremely long for some of the stable organics and inorganics presently allowed into these facilities. Dramatic failures like the Love Canal episode have fueled local public opposition to the development of such facilities; as a result, obtaining a license for a new facility has become very difficult and time consuming. The following factors must be taken into account:

1. *Landfill design.* The design of current-generation perpetual storage chemical landfills takes into account past experience and fail-

ures. These landfills consist of a group of cells dug into the ground, each usually 10 to 30 meters deep and 100 or so meters on a side. Contact between the waste and groundwater is prevented, either by digging the cells into a highly impermeable geological formation such as the clay at the Emmile, Alabama, disposal site or, more commonly, lining the cells with an impermeable barrier. Infiltration into the filled cell by surface water and precipitation is prevented by an impermeable cap placed over the cell when it is filled. The wastes in the landfill are stabilized by segregating them into compatible groups and separating the groups with clay berms that prevent mixing. Dirt fill is forced into any voids between drums or other waste containers and rolled to increase compaction.

Included between the waste and the cell liner is a permeable layer that is designed to collect any leachate that may form and transport it to a sump from which it can be pumped out of the cell. An on-site leachate treatment facility is usually included in the design. Vertical gas collection wells are built in as the waste is placed into the cell, to vent any gas that evolves after the cell is capped. Monitoring wells are dug into the surrounding aquifer, to detect a barrier failure or other problem leading to groundwater contamination. Air monitoring also is required, as is medical surveillance of the operating personnel.

Federal regulations require that a plan be submitted with each application for a new facility, detailing the final closure of the site and demonstrating that adequate financial arrangements will be made for providing funds for implementation. Site closure primarily involves demonstrating the integrity of the cell barriers and landscaping the site so that erosion is minimized. These regulations also require that provisions be made for a 30-year postclosure period, during which the site is to be maintained and monitored.

These new facilities are designed carefully, and their operation is highly regulated.

2.   *Transportation.* Transportation accidents enroute to the landfill can result in an uncontrolled release of waste into the environment. Adequate emergency response and clean-up resources must be available. Surveillance along major routes into the landfill is also advisable, to detect any unreported release. The Department of Transportation regulates the shipment of hazardous waste and requires specific container types and labeling.

3. *Leachate management.* During the cell-filling stage, precipitation introduces water into the cells. Exposed hazardous wastes dissolve or become suspended to some extent, forming a hazardous leachate that must be removed from the cell and treated. Following treatment, the water often is disposed of by evaporation from an unlined spray field, producing potential air-, surface-water-, and groundwater-pollution problems that must be monitored carefully. Over the long term, leachate treatment facilities must be available if it becomes necessary to dewater or recap cells.

4. *Disease control.* As is the case with any complex chemical operation, the potential exists for an on-site disaster that could involve an explosion, a fire, or gas release.ʹEvacuation and disaster response plans must be developed and practiced.

5. *Barrier development.* Most future hazardous chemical waste landfills will require some type of manufactured barrier that will prevent migration of hazardous components from the cell. Polymeric liners and augmented soil liners are under study for their effectiveness as barriers and for their ability to withstand the degradative physical, chemical, and biological processes that may occur. Much remains to be learned about the long-term effectiveness of such barriers. Research is under way to develop techniques for the on-site removal and replacement of a failed liner.

6. *Land use.* Finally, land use of the closed site must be controlled strictly. Any site modifications tending to increase the permeability of the barriers must be avoided, and the possibility of slow evolution of toxic gases or vapors from the cell surfaces must be considered in evaluating any proposed use.

If the use of secure chemical landfills were restricted to treated waste with low leachability, most of the concerns about these facilities would be unnecessary, but with the current broad range of hazardous materials that can be placed into them, a recent EPA comment in its proposed land disposal standards (EPA, 1981) seems quite appropriate:

> While the essential inquiry in evaluating new land disposal facilities will be the acceptability of the facility in protecting human health and the environment, EPA believes that potential applicants should consider managing hazardous waste in a manner that avoids the

necessity of land disposal. As EPA examines the problem of hazard-ous waste management generally, it becomes increasingly convinced that the long-range potential for migration of waste from even the good facilities argues for a long-term strategy that involves phasing out land disposal. However, land disposal remains a necessary op-tion for certain types of hazardous waste at the present time.

Those who manage hazardous waste should at least consider other options (e.g., treatment, recycling and reuse, incineration, and elimination of the materials that generate hazardous waste) before seeking to use land disposal. Such an approach represents sound planning to avoid the long-term responsibility and legal liability (not all of which can be eliminated by complying with an RCRA permit) that will be associated with land disposal in the future.

Regulation of Hazardous Chemical Waste Management

Concern about the disposal of hazardous chemical waste has been expressed in legislation in the United States since the passage of the River and Harbor Act of 1899. Presently, hazardous waste disposal is regulated primarily by Public Law 94-580, the Resource Conservation and Recovery Act (RCRA). This law is discussed in detail in Chapter 8. Regulations promulgated by the EPA, under the authority of RCRA, set criteria and standards for generators and transporters of hazardous waste as well as for facilities for the treatment, storage, and disposal of hazardous waste. A major short-coming of the regulations is a "small quantity exemption" clause that allows generators of a monthly total of less than 1000 kg of most of the hazardous wastes identified to send these wastes to a licensed municipal waste disposal facility. Licensing requirements for such sanitary landfills usually do not require barriers and leachate con-trol systems adequate to protect groundwater and surface water from contamination by highly toxic chemicals. The EPA regulates approx-imately 60,000 generators and estimates that an additional 700,000 generators are excluded under this clause (EPA, 1981).

RCRA provides severe penalties for violators. Conviction of violators can result in penalties of up to $50,000 for each day of the violation and up to two years in prison. Convictions for violations involving "knowing endangerment" (awareness of the potential of death or bodily injury to another person) can result in fines up to

$250,000 and imprisonment for up to five years. The financial liability of a convicted company is limited to $1 million.

Cleanup of Abandoned Waste Sites

In 1980 the Comprehensive Environmental Response, Compensation, and Liability Act, or Superfund, was signed into law. This legislation created a $1.6 billion fund, 85 percent being obtained from a system of taxes on the chemical industry, to be used to finance response to the release of hazardous chemicals into the environment. The principal purpose of the law is to provide an organized response to and funding for dealing with environmental releases of hazardous materials from abandoned or inactive hazardous waste sites. One activity under this legislation is the evaluation of abandoned sites and the establishment of a national priority list containing those sites posing an imminent hazard. These sites then are eligible for cleanup money from the fund. By September 1983, the national priority list contained 546 sites of which five actually had been cleaned up. The legislation requires that parties responsible for a site requiring cleanup pay the associated costs. If they refuse to cooperate, they can be sued for three times the cost of the cleanup and removal of the wastes and the reestablishment of the natural environment.

CASE STUDIES

Minamata

A number of incidents over the past few years have led to the current high level of awareness of the problems associated with hazardous chemical waste management. The case of Minamata, however, represents the classic nightmare of what can happen if management of toxic industrial waste is totally neglected and the waste is allowed to enter the environment directly.

In 1907, a chemical plant was built in Minamata, Japan, a small fishing village on Kyushu Island. In 1932, the plant began producing acetaldehyde, and in the early 1950s production of this chemical was increased greatly. The population of the region grew and prospered as the plant expanded. This developing prosperity did not come without problems, however. The plant was built at the head of Minamata Bay, a small, sheltered inlet of the Shiranui Sea. The plant dumped its wastes into the bay, and the fishermen of the area began to complain of reduced catches shortly after the plant was built. By 1925, the plant was paying the fishermen a small indemnity. In 1950, fish began to float in the bay; in 1952, a variety of land animals and birds began to exhibit unusual behavior. Cats, for example, were observed to salivate, move about with a staggering gait, and suddenly go into convulsions or violently whirl about in circles. By the late 1950s, virtually no cats remained in some parts of Minamata.

In April of 1956, a six-year-old girl with disturbed gait, disturbed speech, and delirium was admitted to the plant hospital. Within five weeks, five more people were admitted with similar symptoms. By 1962, when methyl mercuric chloride was extracted from the plant acetaldehyde sludge, establishing the causative agent in this outbreak of disease, there had been 121 verified human casualties, of which 46 had died. The number of verified victims had risen to 798 by January 1975, with another 2800 suspected cases awaiting verification. At that point the company had paid the equivalent of $80 million in indemnities.

Elizabeth

The pollution control regulations in force in the United States are designed to prevent the type of human and environmental catastrophe that occurred in Minamata. In essence, these regulations are intended to limit the release of most hazardous industrial effluents into the nation's water and air. Clearly, this regulation is necessary, but it has led to the accumulation of vast amounts of hazardous wastes that otherwise would have been dispersed. These materials now must be disposed of in a manner that does not threaten the public health or environment. An incident in Elizabeth, New Jersey, in April 1980 illustrates what can happen if these materials are removed from industrial waste streams but then are allowed to collect without proper disposal.

In the early 1970s the Chemical Control Corporation established a chemical waste storage and disposal facility on the banks of the

Elizabeth River in Elizabeth, New Jersey. In 1977, the New Jersey State Attorney General's Office investigated complaints that Chemical Control was dumping waste into the streets, vacant lots, sewers, and creeks around Newark and Elizabeth. Indictments followed, and the company president was convicted. The new president agreed to inventory the wastes present on the site and to begin appropriate disposal operations. An inspection of the site in January 1979 showed that little progress was being made and that, in fact, deteriorating and leaking drums were stacked four to five deep in many areas over the 50,000-square-foot site. The inspection also uncovered the presence of an astounding array of hazardous materials, including infectious wastes, explosives like picric acid and nitroglycerin, toxins like military nerve gas and cyanides, environmentally stable carcinogens such as polychlorinated biphenyls, and fire and explosion hazards such as benzene and propane gas tanks. By April 1979, state and federal officials had undertaken a cleanup operation at the site. The work was very slow because of the occupational hazards involved and the need to analyze the contents of many containers that were no longer labeled. Fortunately, it was possible to remove many of the most hazardous materials from the site before the night of April 21, 1980, when it was wracked by explosions. Sixty-six persons were injured during the blaze that followed. Emergency plans were made for the evacuation of a portion of Staten Island, but favorable winds directed the toxic plume away from the populated area. Disposal of the debris left on site is an ongoing problem.

The accumulation of hazardous chemical waste at the Chemical Control Corporation site in Elizabeth simply transformed the public health and environmental hazards posed by these wastes from a diffuse problem to an extreme hazard in a localized area. The high population density around the site greatly added to the potential for disaster. Unfortunately, a large number of such uncontrolled "dump sites" exist throughout the United States.

Times Beach

In 1971, a six-year-old girl was hospitalized in St. Louis, Missouri with abdominal pain and blood in her urine. The girl lived on a farm near St. Louis where, earlier that year, 14 horses had begun to bleed from their noses, lose weight, and stagger; seven had died. In addition, hundreds of birds had died on the farm. Similar episodes had occurred on two other nearby farms. At all three farms, the same trucker had been hired earlier in the year to spray horse arenas with waste oil to hold down dust.

Soil samples from the farms were sent to the toxicology lab at the Centers for Disease Control (CDC) in an attempt to identify the responsible toxin. Three years of trial-and-error testing showed that the soil contained 2,3,7,8-TCDD—dioxin (see Chapter 3). The dioxin was traced, through Defense Department records, to a plant in Verona, Missouri that had manufactured Agent Orange for use in Vietnam prior to 1969. In 1969, the plant was leased by Northeast Pharmaceutical and Chemical Company for other purposes, and a company was hired to dispose of remaining chemical wastes. The company subcontracted the job to a trucker named Russell Bliss—the same waste-oil hauler who subsequently sprayed the horse arenas. Bliss, for his part, stated that he did not know that there was dioxin in the oil. Northeast Pharmaceutical later went out of business.

The horse arenas were not the only sites where Bliss had sprayed oil. Another site was Times Beach, a community of 3000 persons on the banks of the Meramec River near St. Louis. In 1972 and 1973, Times Beach had paid Bliss $4900 to spray oil on its gravel roads to control dust. It was nearly 10 years later, however, that the Environmental Protection Agency and the CDC became aware of this fact. Subsequent testing demonstrated that soil samples from Times Beach contained over 100 parts per billion of dioxin—over 100 times the level considered safe.

Just as this information was being made public, the Meramec River flooded, and the residents were forced to evacuate. On the advice of CDC and EPA, the townspeople did not return. EPA purchased the contaminated properties, and Times Beach today stands as a flood-damaged ghost town.

Times Beach was not the only site affected by this episode, however. Perhaps 100 other sites in Missouri and Illinois were sprayed with the dioxin-contaminated oil; investigation of some of these has begun. Altogether, approximately 56 pounds of dioxin were removed from the Verona plant. Less than 14 pounds have been accounted for.

Love Canal

Unlike Elizabeth, New Jersey, it is not certain that Love Canal at Niagara Falls, New York would have become an environmental and public health hazard if appropriate long-term planning, maintenance, and monitoring had been carried out. The details of what occurred, as well as those responsible and liable, still are being contested in the courts and the media (Brown, 1980; Embers, 1980; and Zuesse, 1981).

The story began just before the turn of this century, when an entrepreneur named William T. Love began construction of a sevenmile canal to link the upper and lower levels of the Niagara River near the falls. The project collapsed shortly after it began, leaving only 1000 meters of the canal excavated. In 1942, the Hooker Electrochemical Corporation obtained permission to dispose of its chemical wastes in the canal, and, in 1947, it purchased the canal and 16 acres of land surrounding it.

During the 11 years that Hooker used Love's canal as a burial site, 21,000 tons of waste chemicals were deposited in it, including 6900 tons of Lindane (1,2,3,4,5,6-hexachlorocyclohexane-γ); 2000 tons of chlorobenzenes; 3200 tons of benzoyl and benzylchlorides; and 200 tons of dioxin (see Chapter 3). Hooker chose this site for terminal storage because the area was sparsely populated and the geology of the site would tend to retain the wastes in the canal. Hooker loaded wastes into the north and south ends of the canal in sections isolated by clay berms. As each section was filled, Hooker claims to have covered it with a clay cap 1.2 meters thick, to retain the waste and to prevent surface water infiltration. The geology and structure of the burial cells as reported by Hooker resemble the basic designs and geological requirements for secure chemical landfills in use today.

During the same 11-year period that the canal was used for disposal, the population of the area grew and the demand for land increased. In 1951, the Niagara Falls Board of Education chose the Love Canal property as a location for a school, and there is some evidence (Zuesse, 1981) that pressure was applied to Hooker to relinquish the site. Hooker agreed to donate the property to the school board in 1952. After failing in an attempt to have use of the property restricted to a park, with the school to be built on an adjoining property, Hooker placed provisions in the deed indicating that chemical wastes had been buried on the site and indemnifying itself from any damages or injuries that might result from their presence.

Before the school opened in 1955, the school board approved the removal of 12,900 cubic meters of fill from the canal site. A sanitary sewer, laid three meters below the surface, was cut through the cap and sides of the canal in 1957, and a storm sewer was cut through one side of the canal in 1960. The Board of Education dedicated the northern portion of the canal property to the city in 1960 and sold the southern portion to an individual in 1962. The New York Department of Transportation built an expressway across the southern end of the canal in 1963. During this entire period the surrounding area was developing into a densely populated residential community.

Thus, by 1976, the caps and sides of the trenches had been thinned or breached by fill removal and construction. Heavy rains in 1976 triggered the events that have made Love Canal famous. In October of that year the first reports of chemicals infiltrating nearby basements were received, and an oily black liquid formed pools on top of sections of the canal by late 1977. The State Health Department and the EPA launched a substantial environmental monitoring program that involved obtaining soil samples from the yards of approximately 650 homes and from the landfill itself, air samples, and samples from surface and groundwater in the area and from basement sumps. Analyses of these samples identified the presence of approximately 400 compounds. One of the most alarming findings was 2,3,7,8-tetrachlorodibenzo-2,4-dioxin at 5.3 parts per billion (ppb) in a composite soil sample from the canal site, at 6.7 ppb in a subsurface soil sample from a nearby home, at 30 ppb in sediment samples from an adjoining creek that empties into the Niagara River, and at 3.1 ppb in crayfish taken from this same creek. (In the Times Beach case, the EPA purchased properties from which soil samples were found to contain one ppb or more of dioxin).

In 1978, the state of New York began remedial work at the canal to interrupt the pathways followed by the chemical wastes into the environment, including a tile drainage system and a sloping clay cap. Concurrently, the Governor of New York ordered the permanent relocation of 239 families living in houses immediately adjacent to the canal. In 1980 the federal government designated the

Love Canal neighborhood a disaster area and relocated several hundred more families.

A number of studies then were undertaken to determine if any health effects could be identified in the population and correlated with exposure. An early study indicated a 50-percent increase over the general population in miscarriages in families living around the southern end of the canal. A correlation also was reported between residence along natural drainage features and the incidence of miscarriages, birth defects, and respiratory diseases. In 1980, a study (Kolata, 1980) supported by the EPA reported chromosomal damage in 11 of 36 persons tested. After its release, the study came under serious criticism because of its design.

Recently, Kimbrough, Taylor, Zack, and Heath (1982) reviewed the health-effects studies carried out at Love Canal. They conclude that, with the exception of an early survey study (Vianna, 1980) that suggested reproductive effects, no scientific evidence is available as yet to link exposure to chemicals at Love Canal with health effects. The authors also point out that the population involved is quite small for demonstrating an incidence of disease in excess of that observed in the general population. Also, exposure estimates are very uncertain. In the case of 2,3,7,8-tetrachlorodibenzo-2,4-dioxin, a compound that persists in the human body, an EPA analysis of serum from 36 people from the Love Canal neighborhood failed to demonstrate any exceptional body burden. The controversy over health effects undoubtedly will continue, but the high cost of Love Canal in terms of public funds, psychological trauma, and neighborhood disruption is beyond question.

The episode at Love Canal clearly demonstrates that, if persistent chemicals are to be disposed of by terminal storage in underground cells, long-term maintenance and monitoring are a necessity. Also, utilization of the property after closure of the site must be regulated carefully, to prevent any activity that could breach the barriers designed to prevent migration of the stored wastes.

REFERENCES

Battelle Memorial Institute, Columbus (1981). *Proceedings of the 1981 National Waste Terminal Storage Program Information Meeting.* Washington, D.C.: U.S. Department of Energy, DOE/NWTS-15.

Brown, M. H. (1980). *Laying Waste: The Poisoning of America by Toxic Chemicals*. New York: Pantheon Books.

Eichholz, G. G. (1976). *Environmental Aspects of Nuclear Power*. Ann Arbor, Mich.: Ann Arbor Science Publishers.

Embers, L. R. (1980). Uncertain Science Pushes Love Canal Solutions to Political, Legal Arenas. *Chemical and Engineering News*, August 11, 22–29.

Environmental Protection Agency. (1981). *Hazardous Waste Regulations Under RCRA; A Summary*. Washington, D.C.: EPA SW-939, October.

Epstein, S. S., Brown, L. O., and Pope, C. (1982). *Hazardous Waste in America*. San Francisco: Sierra Club Books.

Johnson, S. A., Warren, J. L., and Lynch, L. (1977). *Financial Analysis of Perpetual Care and Maintenance for the Maxey Flats Low-level Nuclear Waste Disposal Site*. Research Triangle Park, N.C.: Research Triangle Institute, report no. RF23U-1492.

Kimbrough, R. D., Taylor, P. R., Zack, M. M., and Heath, C. W. (1982). Studies of Human Populations Exposed to Environmental Chemicals: Considerations of Love Canal. In *Assessment of Multichemical Contamination: Proceedings of an International Workshop*. Washington, D.C.: National Academy of Sciences.

Kolata, G. B. (1980). Love Canal: False Alarm Caused by Botched Study. *Science*, 208, 1239.

Kovalick, W. W., Jr., Corson, A., Day, H., Dexter, R., Edelman, R., Newton, M., Shannon, M., Strauss, M., and Viviani, D. *State Decision Makers' Guide for Hazardous Waste Management*. Washington, D.C.: U.S. Environmental Protection Agency, EPA SW-612.

Large, D. E. (1981). *Proceedings of the Third Annual Information Meeting DOE Low-Level Waste Management Program*. Washington, D.C.: U.S. Government Printing Office, Oak Ridge National Laboratory report no. ORNL/NFW-81/34.

Legislative Research Commission (1980). *Report of the 1978–1979 Interim Special Advisory Committee on Nuclear Waste Disposal*. Frankfort, Ky.: LRC, Research Report no. 167.

Meyer, G. L. (1976). *Preliminary Data on the Occurrence of Transuranium Nuclides in the Environment at the Radioactive Waste Burial Site, Maxey Flats, Kentucky*. Washington, D.C.: U.S. Government Printing Office, EPA publication no. EPA-520/3-75-021.

Meyer, G. L., Giardina, P. A., DeBonis, M. F., and Eng, J. (1977). *Summary Report on the Low-Level Radioactive Waste Burial Site, West Valley, New York (1963–1975)*. Washington, D.C.: Environmental Protection Agency, EPA-902/4-77-010.

Murphy, E. S., and Holter, G. M. (1980). *Technology, Safety and Costs of Decommission a Reference Low-Level Waste Burial Ground*. Washington, D.C.: U.S. Nuclear Regulatory Commission, NUREG/CR-0570, vols. 1 and 2.

National Institute for Occupational Safety and Health (1981). Formaldehyde: Evidence of Carcinogenicity. *Current Intelligence Bulletin*, 34, April 15.

Rawls, R. L., and O'Sullivan, D. A. (1976). Italy Seeks Answers Following Toxic Release. *Chemical and Engineering News*, August 23, p. 27.

Smith, A. J. (1980). Valley of the Drums, Bullitt County, Kentucky. Washington, D.C.: Environmental Protection Agency, EPA-430/9-80-014.

Sobel, R. (1978). Company Preparedness for RCRA. *Chemecology*, March, 1.

Vianna, N. J., Polan, A. K., Regal, R., Kim, S., Haughie, G. E., and Mitchell, D. (1980). *Adverse Pregnancy Outcomes in the Love Canal Area*. Albany: New York State Department of Health, unpublished report.

Watson, J. E. (1979). *Low-Level Radioactive Waste Management*. Washington, D.C.: Environmental Protection Agency, EPA 520/3-79-002.

Webster, D. A. (1979). Land Burial of Solid Radioactive Waste at Oak Ridge National Laboratory, Tennessee: A Case History. In Carter, Maghossi, and Kahn (eds.), *Management of Low-Level Radioactive Waste*, vol. 2. New York: Pergamon Press.

Zaytsev, V. A. (1982). Development of Low-Waste and Non-Waste Technologies Is the Main Way of Solving the Industrial Waste Problem. Paper presented at the First International Symposium on Environmental Technology for Developing Countries, Bogazici University, Istanbul, Turkey, July 7–14.

Zuesse, E. (1981). Love Canal: The Truth Seeps Out. *Reason*, February, 16–33.

Chapter 8

Environmental
Health Law

*Keith M. Casto**

Environmental health law is that component of environmental law that deals most directly with the impact of environmental contamination on human health.

There are essentially three basic approaches to implementing environmental policy: (1) subsidization, (2) pollution charges, and (3) regulation (Stewart & Krier, 1978). All of these approaches have been employed to some degree, but the regulatory approach is by far the predominant mode in the United States.

Subsidization is a method by which the government would subsidize expenditures for controlling environmental pollution. This approach has been used to a great extent under the Clean Water Act (formerly known as the Federal Water Pollution Control Act) to help defray the cost of sewage treatment. That legislation authorizes the federal government to provide 75 percent matching construction grants for publicly owned sewage treatment plants. Aside from its pollution control aspect in reducing municipal waste water discharge, the construction grants program has been viewed as the largest public works program in history.

---

*This chapter was written by Keith M. Casto in his private capacity. No official support or endorsement by the U.S. Environmental Protection Agency or any other agency of the federal government is intended or should be inferred.

Pollution charges involve the levying of a tax or fee based on the amount of pollution emitted or discharged into the environment. This concept, though popular with academicians, has never been employed fully in the United States. The closest that this approach has ever come to being implemented is the so-called "noncompliance penalty" of the Clean Air Act. Under this provision, any stationary source of air pollution in violation of an applicable emission limitation must pay an administratively assessed penalty based on the economic benefit to that source attributable to the delay in compliance, less a portion of the expenditures made toward compliance.

As indicated, the *regulatory approach* predominates in the United States. The wide acceptance of this approach is reflected in the surprisingly uniform format in which most environmental regulatory legislation is written. The basic framework of the typical environmental regulatory statute can be summarized in terms of goals, standards, legal sanctions, and monitoring authority.

1. *Goals.* Broad, sweeping national environmental goals are enunciated. Examples are " . . . to protect and enhance the quality of the Nation's air resources so as to promote the public health and welfare and the productive capacity of its population" or " . . . it is the national goal that the discharge of pollutants into the navigable waters be eliminated by 1985" or " . . . adequate authority should exist to regulate chemical substances and mixtures which present an unreasonable risk of injury to health or the environment, and to take action with respect to chemical substances and mixtures which are imminent hazards."

2. *Standards.* The statutes typically establish environmental standards (such as national ambient air quality standards, toxic and pretreatment effluent standards, national primary drinking water standards) to be used in implementing goals. Congress casts these generic standards in relatively vague terms: "best available technology economically achievable" or "provides an ample margin of safety" and imposes on the U.S. Environmental Protection Agency (EPA)[1] the responsibility for quantifying these standards. These

---

[1]Established in 1970, the U.S. Environmental Protection Agency is the independent federal regulatory agency responsible for monitoring pollution, developing and enforcing standards, and supporting research in the area of environmental pollution.

generic standards then must be translated into individualized limitations on regulated activities, such as emission or effluent limits for specific pollution sources, restrictions on the use of particular pesticides, limitations on the manufacture of certain chemicals, and so forth.

   3. *Legal sanctions.* The heart of the regulatory approach is the imposition of legal sanctions in the form of civil penalties, administrative seizure or cease-and-desist orders, court injunctions, criminal fines and imprisonment, and, in some cases, debarment from federal contracts, all of which are used to enforce compliance with applicable environmental standards. For purposes of constitutional due process, each statute typically provides for judicial review of environmental regulations in the appropriate United States Court of Appeals. Once upheld by the courts, the regulations routinely become enforceable not only by EPA through the Department of Justice but also by citizens through citizen suit provisions designed to provide an alternative to lax government enforcement as well as an additional incentive to polluters for compliance with applicable requirements.

   4. *Monitoring authority.* All environmental regulatory statutes provide for broad governmental authority to require submission of reports and data and to enter the premises of regulated persons. There are, however, appropriate safeguards to protect trade secrets and other confidential information. In addition, all such statutes confer emergency powers on EPA to act in the event of imminent and substantial risk to public health or the environment.

   With this basic framework in mind, the following seven environmental statutes will be discussed, as they apply to three basic categories of regulation:

1. Regulation from the standpoint of environmental media
   a. The Clean Air Act
   b. The Clean Water Act
   c. The Safe Drinking Water Act
2. Regulation of hazardous substances in the environment
   a. The Resource Conservation and Recovery Act
   b. The Comprehensive Environmental Response, Compensation, and Liability Act

3. Regulation of the production, distribution, and use of pesticides and toxic substances
    a. The Toxic Substances Control Act
    b. The Federal Insecticide, Fungicide, and Rodenticide Act

REGULATION FROM THE STANDPOINT OF ENVIRONMENTAL MEDIA

In this section, we shall discuss three statutes that deal specifically with the *media* that are being protected from pollution (air and water).

Clean Air Act

History and Changing Goals. The primary purpose of the Clean Air Act is "to protect and enhance the quality of the nation's air resources so as to promote the public health and welfare and the productive capacity of its population." To accomplish this, the United States Environmental Protection Agency (EPA) is charged with the responsibility of regulating the emission of air pollutants from both stationary sources of air pollution (coal-fired electric plants, steel mills, copper smelters, incinerators, etc.) and mobile sources (cars, trucks, motorcycles, etc.). Most of our discussion of the Clean Air Act will center on the former – air pollution from stationary sources.

The history of the Clean Air Act reflects an increasing federal presence in the control of a complex and growing problem. The Air Pollution Control Act, passed in 1955, was directed primarily at the support of research, training, and demonstration projects that provided technical assistance to state and local governments upon request. Primary responsibility for the abatement of air pollution fell to the states themselves.

This changed significantly with the passage in 1963 of the Clean Air Act, which authorized the federal government to offer grants to state air pollution control agencies and to intervene legally in efforts to abate interstate air pollution. No concrete substantive goals or "technology-forcing" provisions, however, were designed at that time to achieve the stated goals. The Secretary of the Department of Health, Education and Welfare did establish air quality criteria based on scientific knowledge of the effects of various concentrations of certain air pollutants, which formed the basis for the establishment of standards later on.

The 1967 Air Quality Act was the first step toward a distinctly regulatory approach, as exemplified in its premise that "the prevention and control of air pollution at its source is the primary responsibility of states and local governments." It required states to establish, adopt, and submit "ambient air quality standards" for "air quality control regions" within those states. The 1970 and 1977 amendments reflect a full-fledged effort to establish a comprehensive, technology-forcing, enforcement oriented regulatory scheme with strong legal sanctions and an overriding, if not predominant, federal presence.

These amendments address themselves specifically to three separate categories of stationary sources of air pollution: existing sources, new sources, and hazardous air pollutants.

National Ambient Air Quality Standards (NAAQS).   For existing sources of air pollution, the NAAQS—required by the 1970 amendment—were designed to provide minimal standards nationwide for protecting public health and welfare. "Primary" NAAQS are designed to protect public health with an adequate margin of safety; "secondary" NAAQS are designed to protect public welfare (i.e., property, aesthetics). Ambient air quality standards have been established for particulate matter, sulfur oxides, nitrogen oxides, carbon monoxide, photochemical oxidant/hydrocarbon, and lead (see Chapter 5). In addition, the EPA is required to investigate the need for ambient standards for radioactive pollutants, cadmium, arsenic, and polycyclic organic matter.

The Clean Air Act Amendments of 1970 and 1977 insist that the states take primary responsibility for attaining and maintaining these standards. The actual standards to be achieved, however, are nationally uniform, not geopolitically diverse according to state. Each state must submit to the EPA a "state implementation plan" for the attainment of NAAQS, within certain legally mandatory deadlines set forth in the act. The state implementation plan for each pollutant for which an ambient air quality standard has been established must include legally enforceable source-specific limitations, the cumulative effect of which is to attain and maintain air quality standards.

New-source Performance Standards (NSPS). The standards set in this 1970 amendment are direct technology-forcing provisions that set specific emission limitations for certain industrial categories of specific sources. These standards, too, are nationally uniform. This means that if the best air pollution control technology is available on a pilot plant basis (as opposed to a full-scale operation basis), the new-source performance standard can be established with respect to that technology. Each standard "reflects the degree of emission reduction which the Administrator determines has been adequately demonstrated for that category of sources." The effect of this regulation is to motivate the development of pilot projects into full-scale operations. At the same time, the EPA has attempted to provide financial incentives for the development of pilot projects, through grants administered by its office of research and development.

National Emission Standards for Hazardous Air Pollutants (NESHAPS). In 1977, the EPA was authorized to set nationally uniform standards for both new and existing sources of designated hazardous air pollutants, defined in Section 112 of the Clean Air Act as

> . . . an air pollutant to which no ambient air quality standard is applicable and which in the judgment of the Administrator causes, or contributes to, air pollution which may reasonably be anticipated to result in an increase in serious irreversible, or incapacitating reversible, illness.

The pollutants for which standards have been set are beryllium, asbestos, mercury, and vinyl chloride. The EPA also has listed inorganic arsenic, radionuclides, and benzene as hazardous air pollutants, but no control standards have been established. The EPA also has indicated an intent to list acrylonitrile, formaldehyde, nickel, and polycyclic organic matter in the near future.

The 1977 amendments codify EPA's earlier position that the Clean Air Act prohibits the use of dispersion techniques such as tall stacks and intermittent controls—such as production restrictions based on adverse meteorological conditions—as permanent control methods in order to achieve and maintain ambient air quality standards. Continuous emission controls such as low-sulfur fuels and flue gas scrubbers are specifically required as permanent control methods.

Deadlines and Litigation. Under the state implementation plans submitted pursuant to the 1970 Clean Air Act amendments, all states were to have attained the primary (i.e., public health) standards by July 1, 1975, except for a few areas granted an extension to mid 1977. Secondary (i.e., public welfare) standards were to have been attained within a "reasonable time"; in many states this was the same date as for primary standards attainment. The 1977 amendments extended the primary standards deadline to the end of 1982 (with an additional extension — to the end of 1987 — for photochemical oxidants and carbon monoxide, in some cases).

In 1976, in the case of Union Electric *v.* EPA (421 U.S. 426), the Supreme Court held that the EPA is not authorized by the act to disapprove state implementation plans on the grounds that they are economically or technologically infeasible, as long as the plans are sufficient for attaining and maintaining ambient standards. This is a decided change from the preexisting law, which allowed air pollution sources to avoid compliance when it could be shown that abatement of the pollution was technologically and economically infeasible. The ambient air quality standards thus can be viewed as significant, though indirect, provisions authorizing "technology-forcing," which was one of the primary goals of the 1970 amendments.

The 1970 amendments, literally read, would have prevented the siting of any new sources of air pollution in areas where ambient air quality standards were not achieved, thus preventing virtually all growth in those areas. Consequently, the phase-out of older, dirtier existing technology in favor of newer, cleaner technology would tend to be stifled because the act would prevent any replacement in and around heavily industrialized nonattainment areas. Therefore, a nonattainment policy — called the "offset" policy — was adopted in 1976 to allow new growth in these areas only if stringent conditions were met. These conditions were designed to reduce new-source emissions to the greatest degree possible, in order to obtain more than equivalent emission reductions (i.e., "offsets") from existing sources and to achieve a net air quality benefit.

Environmental public interest groups forced the EPA, through federal court litigation, to take steps to prevent significant deterioration of air quality in areas that were relatively cleaner than nonattainment areas. As a result, the EPA adopted regulations on December 5, 1974 designed to achieve this result. The program was implemented through a preconstruction and premodification review process for certain specific categories of stationary sources of air pollution. The process was designed to prevent the construction of new sources or major modification of existing sources that would cause significant deterioration of air quality. The 1977 amendments statutorily legitimized this Prevention of Significant Deterioration (PSD) program, with certain modifications that made it more stringent and comprehensive.

Enforcement Sanctions and Violations.   The 1977 amendments, which essentially incorporated the "offset" policy, were to be replaced by revised state implementation plans by July 1, 1979. The sanction for not having an EPA-approved plan revision for an area designated nonattainment by July 1, 1979 was that no major new sources of air pollution could be constructed or modified in that area.

Currently the Clean Air Act provides a broad array of enforcement sanctions for violations of applicable requirements, including the following:

1. Judicially imposed civil penalties of $25,000 per day of violation
2. Injunctive relief (a court order requiring compliance)
3. Administrative orders (orders issued by EPA requiring compliance)
4. Criminal penalties of $25,000 per day of violation and/or imprisonment of up to one year for the first conviction; $50,000 per day and imprisonment of up to two years for any subsequent conviction
5. Automatic administratively assessed noncompliance penalties based upon the economic value of noncompliance
6. Debarment from federal procurement contracts

Mobile Sources of Air Pollution.   Of the potential mobile sources of air pollution, Title II of the Clean Air Act regulates only those vehicles that travel our nation's highways: automobiles, trucks, buses, and motorcycles. According to the National Commission on Air Quality's report in March 1981, the exhaust from these vehicles makes the largest contribution to air pollution in the country (34% of hydrocarbons, 75% of carbon monoxide, and 29% of nitrogen oxides).

The Clean Air Act establishes a number of mechanisms for regulating emissions from these sources. The pivotal mechanism is the bundle of emission limitations on hydrocarbon, carbon monoxide, and nitrogen oxide from the vehicles themselves. The act also provides that emission limits for other pollutants may be established if the data show that they cause or contribute to adverse health or welfare effects. In addition, the act requires the EPA to establish emission standards for particulates.

Manufacturers may obtain waivers of the vehicle emission standards on a case-by-case basis. As of March 1981, the EPA had granted waivers to approximately 30 percent of the 1981 and 1982 model year automobiles for carbon monoxide and to all 1981 and most 1982 diesel vehicles for the nitrogen oxides standard.

The EPA also has promulgated emission standards for evaporative hydrocarbon emissions from gasoline automobiles and light trucks, beginning with the 1971 model year, and for heavy gasoline trucks, beginning in the 1982 model year.

Before a manufacturer can offer a vehicle for sale, the EPA must issue a certificate of conformity. To obtain certification, a manufacturer must submit several prototype vehicles of each engine family to the EPA for testing. The EPA is authorized by the Clean Air Act to conduct, or to require manufacturers to conduct, any tests necessary to ensure compliance with the emission standards. In addition, the EPA is authorized to test production vehicles upon leaving the assembly line. If 40 percent or more of these vehicles do not comply with the emissions standards, the EPA can revoke or suspend the certificate of conformity issued on the basis of the prototype testing. The EPA also may order the recall of any class of vehicles, if a substantial number of them do not comply with the standards throughout their useful life because of defective vehicle design or manufacture.

The manufacturer of a new motor vehicle must provide the purchaser with a warranty that covers the design and crafting of components that affect the level of exhaust emissions. This warranty remains in effect for the useful life of the vehicle (i.e., five years or 50,000 miles). There is also a two-year or 24,000-mile manufacturer's warranty that covers the failure of a vehicle to pass a state inspection and maintenance program.

Section 211 of the Clean Air Act governs the regulation of lead and other additives used in gasoline. Under this section, the EPA has required fuel refiners, producers, distributors, and service stations to make available unleaded gasoline, which must be used in all vehicles equipped with catalytic converters. This serves two purposes: to reduce lead emissions and to prevent impairment of the effectiveness of catalytic converters.

The act also requires that states implement inspection and maintenance programs in areas that did achieve compliance with the photochemical oxidant/hydrocarbon or carbon monoxide ambient air quality standards by 1982. These programs are intended to insure that in-use vehicles comply with applicable emissions standards.

Clean Water Act

The Clean Water Act, like the Clean Air Act, is the product of incremental legislation over a considerable period of time, which resulted in an increasingly dominant federal role. It began as the Federal Water Pollution Control Act (FWPCA) in 1948 and was amended five times before it was rewritten comprehensively in 1972 with a distinctly technology-forcing, enforcement oriented, federal regulatory approach.

History and Purpose. The 1965 amendments established state water quality standards for intrastate waters. The cumbersome process established to implement this legislation proved time consuming and ineffective. In 1970, the government implemented a section that prohibited the discharge of "refuse" into navigable waters without a permit from the Secretary of the Army. This Refuse Act Permit Program remained in force until 1972, when the FWPCA was substantially revised. It was amended again in 1977 to relax some of the requirements in the act when it appeared that certain deadlines would not be met by a large number of sources and to shift the focus of the act from conventional water pollutants (such as total suspended solids, pH, biological oxygen demand) to toxic pollutants. At this time, the FWPCA also was renamed the Clean Water Act. Its purpose, in summary, was (1) to provide federal financial assistance for the construction of publicly owned sewage treatment plants; (2) to regulate the discharge of pollutants from point sources; and (3) to regulate spills of oil and hazardous substances.

The 1972 Amendments: NPDES. The standards established under the National Pollutant Discharge Elimination System (NPDES) formed the heart of the 1972 amendments. The system was designed to make all of our waters fishable and swimmable by 1983 and to eliminate the discharge of all pollutants by 1985. These amendments introduced technology-forcing effluent standards, that is, the quantifiable limit of a particular pollutant that may be discharged by a specific source ("point source") in a given time period. Effluent standards apply to both industrial and publicly owned (e.g., municipal sewage treatment plants) sources.

A permit issued to each "point source" contains specific effluent limitations, compliance schedules for meeting those limits (with interim increments of progress), and reporting and monitoring requirements.

Under Section 301 of the 1972 act, all sources directly discharging into surface waters were required to meet increasingly stringent technology-based effluent limitations in two distinct phases: the less stringent level by July 1, 1977 and the more stringent level by July 1, 1983.

These amendments maintained the basic structure of state-set and EPA-approved water quality standards and expanded the reach of these standards to include interstate as well as intrastate waters.

The 1977 Amendments: Delays, Modification, Litigation. The Clean Water Act of 1977 extended the 1977 deadline for industrial dischargers to April 1, 1979, if certain stringent conditions were met. The 1977 requirements for publicly owned treatment works (POTWs) were extended to 1983, if their noncompliance was caused by unavoidable construction delays or lack of federal funds.

There were other revisions as well. Requirements for control of conventional pollutants were modified to allow much greater consideration of the costs of complying with these standards. The standard of "best available technology" (BAT) was relaxed to become "best conventional technology" (BCT). In addition, the focus shifted from the control of conventional pollutants to an emphasis on toxic pollutants, which, it was realized, represent a much greater environmental threat.

Standards for Toxic Pollutants. Section 307(a) of the Clean Water Act requires the EPA to set effluent standards for toxic pollutants. The toxic effluent standards must provide for "an ample margin of safety." The act specifically states that the effluent standard may take the form of a "prohibition." This is based on the act's enunciated "national policy that the discharge of toxic pollutants in toxic amounts be prohibited." The standards themselves had to be achieved within one year of promulgation.

Standards for Pretreatment. An industrial discharger may prefer, for economic or other reasons, to discharge into publicly owned treatment works rather than directly into water courses. In such a case the publicly owned treatment plant becomes the discharger rather than the particular industry that ties into that plant. Because the quality of the effluent from the publicly owned treatment plant often is affected substantially by the nature and quantity of the influent from the industrial discharger, restrictions must be placed on the industrial influent in order to protect the operation of the treatment plant from pollutants that may interfere with various treatment processes. These standards for pretreatment are established under Section 307(b) of the Clean Water Act (Rogers, 1977).

Dischargers into municipal treatment works are not required to have an NPDES permit; however, the treatment works must obtain a permit for any discharge.

Other Types of Pollution Standards. The Clean Water Act subjects thermal pollution — caused primarily by the use of cooling water by electric power plants — to the same nationally uniform technology-based standards as any other pollution. It also establishes a separate permit program for the discharge of dredged or fill material into navigable waters. Dredge and fill permits are issued by the Secretary of the Army (through the Corps of Engineers) with the concurrence of the EPA. In addition, the Clean Water Act prohibits discharges of oil or hazardous substances into "navigable waters of the United States, adjoining shorelines, or into or upon the waters of the contiguous zone."

Enforcement of Standards. A federal permit system was established under Section 402 of the Clean Water Act, to enforce the effluent and water quality standards applicable to direct discharges into surface water. Discharge of any pollutant into waters of the United States without a permit, or discharge in violation of the conditions of any permit, is unlawful and gives rise to the enforcement of sanctions available under the act.

Against the backdrop of the strong language prohibiting the discharge of toxic pollutants in Section 307(a) — as discussed previously — the Clean Water Act and its complex legislative history create uncertainty as to whether or not the EPA could consider the availability of control technology in setting these standards.

This uncertainty, coupled with the unrealistic time frame for compliance, resulted in delay by the EPA in the issuance of standards, as well as protracted administrative proceedings by industrial dischargers challenging the standards for additional pollutants on a more expeditious basis. This forced the EPA to shift its focus toward the more conventional approach of using technology-based standards to achieve as much control of toxic pollutants as technologically feasible by including toxic substances in the 1983 BAT standards for individual industries. This necessarily injected greater consideration of costs and technological availability into the formulation of the standards, contrary to the congressional mandate in 1972. The culmination of this effort was a settlement agreement with several environmental organizations, committing the EPA to a schedule for promulgating BAT effluent standards for 21 major industries and for 65 (and ultimately expanded to 129) "priority pollutants" with toxic characteristics.

The 1977 amendments to the Clean Water Act specifically ratify this agreement and incorporate certain changes to make this section easier to implement (e.g., allowing industries up to three years to comply if the one-year deadline is technologically infeasible). To date, the EPA has fallen substantially behind schedule in the promulgation of these toxic standards because of the inherently complex task of formulating precise standards for particular toxic pollutants based on the technology available in diverse industries.

In the case of dischargers into municipal treatment works, violations of the permit are enforceable by the treatment works, by the

EPA, or by the state to which the permit program has been delegated, and action may be brought to restrain or prohibit any new tie-ins to the treatment works.

The Future.   As more information becomes available regarding the environmental impact and disposition of water pollutants (particularly toxic pollutants), the use of water quality standards in the formulation of permit limits will become increasingly important. This means that the states will tend to have a greater role in the regulation of water pollution in the future, since the act does not preclude state water-quality-based requirements that are at least as stringent as the federal technology-based requirements.

Finally, Section 201(c) of the Clean Water Act provides for waste treatment management to be done, to the extent practicable, on an areawide basis and to "provide control or treatment of all point and nonpoint sources of pollution, including in-place or accumulated pollution sources. To accomplish this, the act provides for federal grants to state, local, and regional agencies for treatment works. The federal share of these construction grants is 75 percent of the construction costs of the treatment works. This program represents the largest public works program in the history of the federal government.

Safe Drinking Water Act

The Safe Drinking Water Act (SDWA), which became effective December 1, 1974, provides for national drinking water regulations for public water systems, that is, systems for piped water for *human* consumption that have at least 15 service connections or regularly serve at least 25 individuals.

Regulations.   These regulations are required to identify contaminants that may have adverse human health effects and specify maximum contaminant levels (MCLs) for each of the contaminants so identified. The contaminants for which MCLs have been established are arsenic; barium; cadmium; chromium; lead; mercury; selenium; silver; endrin; lindane; methoxychlor; toxaphene; 2,4-D; 2,4,5-TP; Silvex; trihalomethanes; nitrates; coliform bacteria; fluoride; turbidity; and radionuclides.

The regulations are divided into primary and secondary regulations. Primary drinking water regulations are designed to protect humans from adverse health effects. The secondary drinking water regulations are designed to protect public welfare and specify maximum contaminant levels for such items as taste, odor, color, appearance, or anything that might cause the public to discontinue use of that water or otherwise adversely affect public welfare. These secondary levels represent reasonable goals for drinking water quality but are not federally enforceable. They are intended as discretionary guidelines for the states; however, the states may establish higher or lower levels as appropriate to their particular circumstances. These regulations are further subdivided into interim and revised drinking water regulations. Although the interim drinking water regulations went into effect in 1977, the revised drinking water regulations have not yet been published.

Within one year of the effective date of the statute, the EPA was to have proposed and promulgated regulations to prevent the underground injection of chemical wastes and other materials that endanger drinking water sources. The regulations were promulgated on June 24, 1980 and became effective on July 24, 1980.

Enforcement.   Under Section 1413 of the act, a state (rather than the EPA) can have primary enforcement authority if it is determined by the EPA that the state has adopted regulations no less stringent than the National Primary Drinking Water Regulations and is adequately enforcing those regulations.

If a state to which primary enforcement responsibility has been delegated fails to bring a noncomplying system into compliance, the EPA may bring suit in federal district court to compel compliance.

Each owner or operator of a public water system must give notice to the persons served by it of any failure on the part of the system to comply with a national primary drinking water regulation.

VARIANCES.   The law also provides for variances from National Primary Drinking Water Regulations where the raw water quality makes it impossible to meet maximum contaminant levels, despite application of best technology, treatment techniques, or other means that are "generally available (taking costs into consideration)." These variances must include a schedule for compliance; however, very few variances have been granted and they related only to new water supplies.

EXEMPTIONS.   A state that has primary enforcement responsibility may grant to any public water supply system an exemption from any MCL or treatment technique upon a finding that:

1. Due to compelling factors the utility cannot comply
2. The system was in operation on the effective date of such regulation, or, for a system not in operation by that date, only if no reasonable alternative source of drinking water is available to such system
3. The granting of such exemption will not result in an unreasonable health risk

Under this section, a compliance and implementation schedule must be established. To date, relatively few exemptions have been granted.

EMERGENCY POWERS AND SNARLS. Under Section 1431, the EPA (notwithstanding any other provision in the act) upon receipt of information that a contaminant that is present in or likely to enter a public water system may present an imminent and substantial endangerment to human health, may take such action as is deemed necessary in order to protect human health. The EPA also must find, however, that the appropriate state and local authorities have not acted in a timely or appropriate manner. The EPA then may issue administrative orders or commence a civil action for injunctive relief. Willful violations of any order issued by the EPA under this section can result in fines of up to $5,000 per day of violation. This section has been used in hazardous waste cases along with comparable provisions in the Clean Water Act and the Resource Conservation and Recovery Act (RCRA; discussed later). The most notable example is the Love Canal/Hooker Chemical litigation in New York.

"Suggested No Adverse Response Levels" (SNARLS) have been developed administratively by the EPA to provide guidance to regional offices and the states as to the levels of selective contaminants, not previously covered by MCLs in a public drinking system, at which the risk of endangerment to public health is sufficiently elevated so as to advise the public not to drink the water. These levels have no legal effect but are advisory only. The EPA has been using these levels as guidelines in determining when there is an imminent and substantial endangerment to human health, for purposes of the exercise of emergency powers under the Safe Drinking Water Act and RCRA.

REGULATION OF HAZARDOUS SUBSTANCES IN THE ENVIRONMENT

Resource Conservation and Recovery Act

History and Purpose.   The Resource Conservation and Recovery Act of 1976 (RCRA) is actually an amendment to the Solid Waste Disposal Act of 1965, which has been amended on three other occasions: in 1970 by the Resource Recovery Act, in 1978 by the Quiet Communities Act, and in 1980 by the Solid Waste Disposal Act Amendments of 1980. However, the act continues to be referred to commonly as RCRA.

RCRA is designed to fill in the gaps not covered by other federal environmental regulatory legislation. In a sense, the Clean Air Act and the Clean Water Act attempt to regulate waste (in the form of pollution) in distinct media — the air and the water. This media-oriented legislation, however, does not regulate directly much of our air and water pollution that is caused by the intentional treatment, storage, transportation, and disposal of waste, particularly hazardous waste. For example, the Clean Air Act regulates only a handful of hazardous air pollutants and the Clean Water Act generally does not regulate waste that leaches into and contaminates groundwater. RCRA, on the other hand, attempts to regulate the problem of waste, irrespective of the receiving medium for such wastes.

By definition, RCRA regulates only "solid waste"; however, the term is defined so broadly under the act [Section 104(27)] as to include, with certain specific exceptions, all waste except uncontained gaseous material. The word "solid" in the term "solid waste" is therefore meaningless because of its expansive definition. The most important subset of this definition from an environmental health standpoint is "hazardous waste," which is defined as

a solid waste, or combination of solid wastes, which because of its quantity, concentration, or physical, chemical, or infectious characteristics may—(A) cause, or significantly contribute to an increase in mortality or an increase in serious irreversible, or incapacitating reversible, illness; or (B) pose a substantial present or potential hazard to human health or the environment when improperly treated, stored, transported, or disposed of, or otherwise managed.

Only that part of RCRA which deals with hazardous waste management will be discussed, because those other provisions of the act that relate to the disposal of municipal solid waste and resource recovery do not relate substantially to environmental health.

Regulatory Scheme.   Congress responded to the problem of improper disposal of hazardous waste by constructing a somewhat complex "cradle-to-grave" management system, with the emphasis placed on the proper management of hazardous waste rather than on the reduction in the generation of such waste. This approach requires the tracking of hazardous wastes from the point of generation until final disposal by means of a manifest record-keeping and reporting system with positive controls on treatment, storage, and disposal facilities.

Identification and Listing of Hazardous Waste.   The EPA was required by the RCRA to establish the criteria for specific identification and listing of hazardous wastes. The agency then used these criteria to establish a list of hazardous wastes by specific wastes, waste sources, and waste processes, and to establish characteristics for identifying additional hazardous wastes. These characteristics were developed on the basis of the availability of standardized tests or the opportunity for reasonable detection by generators, through their knowledge of the waste.

The four characteristics established were: (1) ignitability (capable of causing or exacerbating fires); (2) corrosivity (causes harm to human tissue, promotes migration of toxic contaminants from other wastes, reacts dangerously with other wastes, harms aquatic life, and corrodes metal containers); (3) reactivity (tendency to explode or react violently); and (4) toxicity.

Anyone who generates, transports, treats, stores, or disposes of hazardous waste is required to notify the EPA. Upon submission of this notification, the EPA provides each notifier with an identification number to be used for purposes of tracking hazardous waste, under the manifest system.

The Tracking System. The generator is the most important participant in the tracking system. The generator must determine if the waste generated is hazardous. If so, the hazardous waste must be appropriately containerized (with proper labeling and marking) and a manifest (shipping form) must be prepared that will insure that the waste arrives at its intended destination, if the waste is treated, stored, or disposed of at some location other than the generator's property. The generator must keep records of all shipments and report any shipments to the EPA (or the state regulatory agency, if the federal program is delegated to that state) that do not reach the facility designated on the manifest. In this way, the generator remains ultimately liable for appropriate disposition of the waste, and that responsibility cannot be shifted to another by contract.

The EPA and the Department of Transportation (DOT) jointly regulate the transportation of hazardous waste. Under the regulations, the transporter must have an EPA identification number; deliver all hazardous waste to the designated treatment, storage, or disposal facility; and comply with the EPA manifest requirements for tracking and transporting hazardous waste. The transporter must comply also with DOT requirements regarding the reporting of spills or discharges and must clean up any wastes discharged during transportation.

Permits for Treatment, Storage, and Disposal. Facilities such as landfills, incinerators, tanks, surface impoundments, and drum storage areas that treat, store, or dispose of hazardous wastes (Treatment, Storage, and Disposal Facilities, or TSDFs) may operate only with a permit or "interim status." This is a grandfather mechanism that allows waste to be disposed of in certain existing facilities until those facilities are issued RCRA permits under more stringent standards and conditions.

RCRA permits the EPA to delegate the operation of the federal hazardous waste program to the states under a two-phased authorization. States that have programs substantially equivalent to the federal program may receive "interim authorization" until such programs can qualify for the second and final phase, "final authorization."

Exemptions. The definition of solid waste under the current regulations includes materials that are not always discarded and thus may include materials that are used, reused, reclaimed, or recycled. Therefore, the materials also are regulated under this system, since they pose a danger to health or the environment, whether they are destined for disposal or recycling. However, the EPA has sought deliberately to reduce the regulatory burdens on handlers of recycled waste in order to stimulate recycling activity.

In addition, certain wastes are excluded from regulation under RCRA: (1) domestic sewage; (2) industrial waste water discharges; (3) nuclear wastes regulated under the Atomic Energy Act; (4) irrigation return flows; (5) household wastes; (6) agricultural and silvicultural wastes returned to the soil as fertilizers or conditioners; (7) mining wastes; (8) waste generated by combustion of fossil fuels; (9) wastes associated with exploration, development, or production of crude oil, natural gas, or geothermal energy; and (10) used, reused, recycled, or reclaimed hazardous waste that is not a sludge or is identified only by characteristic. Also exempted are small generators who generate less than 1000 kg of hazardous waste per month, except for certain acutely hazardous wastes for which lower levels have been set.

Scope of the Problem: Mismanagement Then and Now.   The EPA estimated in 1980 that at least 57 million metric tons of the total wasteload of the United States were classified as hazardous. "These wastes range in nature from common household trash to complex materials in industrial wastes, sewage, sludge, agricultural residues, mining refuse, and pathological waste from institutions such as hospitals and laboratories" (EPA, 1980, p. 1). Approximately 90 percent of this waste has been disposed of by environmentally unsafe methods, such as unlined surface impoundments, improperly sited or managed land disposal, and uncontrolled incineration. The chemical industry (e.g., plastics, synthetic fibers, fertilizers, pesticides, synthetic rubber, paints, pigments, medicines, soaps, detergents, cosmetics, explosives, adhesives) generates approximately 50 percent of industrial hazardous waste. About 60 percent of this waste is generated in 10 states: New Jersey, Illinois, Ohio, California, Pennsylvania, Texas, New York, Michigan, Tennessee, and Indiana. The number of uncontrolled hazardous waste sites has been estimated to be 9650, as of June 30, 1981, according to the EPA Hazardous Waste Site Tracking System.

Violation and Enforcement.   The most egregious form of hazardous waste mismanagement is the transfer of such waste by supposedly reputable companies to questionable transporters (the so-called "midnight dumpers") for disposal, with no control by the generators of the waste over either the destination or the method of disposal. Congress's response to the problem has been to emphasize proper management of hazardous waste, as in the tracking system described previously, rather than to reduce the generation of such waste. Although RCRA was enacted in 1976, the scope of the problem was not appreciated fully until August 1978, when President Carter declared a state of emergency in the residential area of Niagara Falls, New York—the Love Canal—where approximately 21,000 tons of industrial wastes had been deposited by Hooker Chemicals and Plastics Corporation between 1942 and 1953 (see Chapter 7).

Such mismanagement of hazardous waste is attributable to the strong economic incentives for avoiding the cost and complexity of environmentally acceptable methods of disposal, and to the lack of technological expertise that appropriate management requires. However, the current regulatory burdens on waste handlers will tend to stimulate the seeking of alternatives to generating hazardous waste as well as opportunities for recycling such waste.

Subtitle C of RCRA governs only the ongoing management of hazardous waste after November 19, 1980. Section 7003 of RCRA provides that the federal government may bring suit against any person (including a generator) who contributes to the handling, storage, treatment, transportation, or disposal of hazardous or solid waste that may present an imminent and substantial endangerment to health or the environment. This allows a federal district court to require cleanup of hazardous waste sites, such as Love Canal, that became inactive before the effective date of the RCRA regulations. In addition, the Administrator of the EPA may issue administrative orders to effect the same purpose. This section has been used by the EPA and the Department of Justice to effect cleanup of dozens of sites all over the country.

The major problem with the use of this authority is the difficulty in finding financially responsible defendants to perform the necessary remedial action. Congress responded to this problem by enacting the Comprehensive Environmental Response, Compensation, and Liability Act of 1980, also known as "Superfund."

The Comprehensive Environmental Response, Compensation, and Liability Act of 1980 ("Superfund")

History and Purpose.   The 1970s often are called "the Environmental Decade" because of the extensive number of statutes passed by Congress during that decade in an attempt to deal with our most obvious and pressing environmental problems. This massive regulatory effort has raised the public awareness about environmental pollution and thereby increased our sophistication in recognizing environmental problems (such as those caused by abandoned hazardous waste sites) and in appreciating their potential effects on human health.

The consequences of this enhanced public (and professional) sensitivity have been fourfold: (1) the identification of additional and more disturbing environmental problems; (2) growing dissatisfaction by regulated industry with the extent and complexity of governmental regulation in the environmental area; (3) the increased assertion of private legal rights for compensation for harm caused by environmental contamination resulting in protracted, complex, and often indecisive and unsuccessful litigation; and (4) the realization that perhaps the rate of discovery of hazardous environmental problems is outstripping our collective ability to solve or even control them through piecemeal governmental regulation.

More than 20 bills were introduced during the 96th Congress (1978–1980) to deal comprehensively with all forms of toxic environmental pollution in a manner that would reduce reliance on a complex environmental regulatory scheme and expedite remedial action and compensation for victims. What emerged was a compromise piece of legislation signed into law on December 11, 1980, entitled the Comprehensive Environmental Response, Compensation, and Liability Act of 1980 and commonly referred to as "Superfund." Superfund is essentially a remedial action measure whose liability aspect is limited to reimbursement for cleanup. Restoration of property with compensation for personal injury is left to traditional common-law remedies.

"Superfund" is so named because the predominant feature of the legislation is its creation of a Hazardous Substances Response Fund to effect cleanup and remedial action whenever there is a release of a hazardous substance that presents a real or potential threat to public health. There is no need to initiate legal action first against the responsible party or parties. The fund consists of $1.6 billion financed over a five-year period by fees levied on petroleum and selected industrial chemicals (87.5% or $1.38 billion), with the balance financed by general tax revenues (12.5% or $220 million).

Central to the use and operation of the fund is the concept of a "release" of a "hazardous substance." A "release" is broadly defined but excludes occupational exposure, most engine exhaust emissions, releases of radioactive materials during a "nuclear accident," the "normal" application of fertilizer, and releases permitted under other federal environmental regulatory statutes.

Utilization of the Fund. The act authorizes the President of the United States to utilize the fund to take removal and remedial action whenever there is an actual or threatened release into the environment of a "hazardous substance" or "any pollutant or contaminant which may present an imminent and substantial danger to the public health or welfare. . . . " The governmental response actions are limited to a time period of six months or to the expenditure of $1 million, whichever occurs first, except in certain emergencies or where the state in which the release occurs enters into a contract or cooperative agreement for the sharing of response costs and responsibilities.

Governmental discovery of actionable releases is intended to be accomplished through a comprehensive mandatory reporting scheme with stiff sanctions for failure to notify. First, Section 102 of the act requires the EPA to designate a list of hazardous substances and to establish reportable quantities for such substances. Section 103 of Superfund requires that, in the event of a release of a reportable quantity of a hazardous substance from a vessel or facility, the person responsible for that vessel or facility must immediately notify the National Response Center established under the Clean Water Act. Second, owners or operators of facilities at which hazardous substances have been stored, treated, or disposed, and transporters of hazardous substances to such facilities, were required to notify the EPA of the existence of such facilities on or before June 9, 1981.

Abatement Action and Enforcement of Cleanups. Whenever there may be "an imminent and substantial endangerment to the public health or welfare or the environment because of an actual or threatened release of a hazardous substance from a facility," the government may bring an action in federal district court to seek abatement of such danger or threat or such other action as may be appropriate. The president also may take other appropriate action, including the issuance of orders to protect public health and welfare or the environment, the violation of which will subject the violator to fines up to $5,000 per day. In addition, failure to provide the remedial action required by the president may subject the responsible party to punitive damages of up to three times the amount of any response costs incurred by the fund.

Any person who is responsible for the release of a hazardous substance that gives rise to the incurrence of response costs is liable for such costs. Aside from certain specified limited defenses, liability attaches without regard to fault (i.e., strict liability).

The act eliminated virtually all private claims for compensation. The effect of this limitation is to defer resolution of the controversial issue of creating a fund for compensating the personal injuries of victims of environmental harm.

Subtitle C of the act creates a special fund for purposes of cleaning up hazardous waste facilities that have been issued permits under RCRA and have been closed in accordance with RCRA permit requirements. This fund, which will not exceed $200 million, will be financed by a tax of $2.13 per dry weight ton of hazardous waste on permitted hazardous waste facilities.

REGULATION OF THE PRODUCTION, DISTRIBUTION AND USE OF PESTICIDES AND TOXIC SUBSTANCES

The Toxic Substances Control Act of 1976 (TSCA)

History and Purpose.   Since World War II, this country has experienced a proliferation of synthetic organic chemicals. It is estimated that there are currently 50,000 or more types of chemicals in commerce, with approximately 1000 new ones being introduced every year (Jennings, 1981). Prior to 1976, chemical manufacturers (other than pesticide manufacturers) had never been required to evaluate newly marketed chemicals for health risks.

After several years of substantial debate, TSCA was enacted in 1976. The act takes essentially a two-pronged approach: (1) to regulate those chemicals currently in existence that may be "imminently hazardous" and (2) to prevent new chemicals from entering the market that may present "an unreasonable risk of injury to health or the environment (Druly & Ordway, 1977). The act thus takes a different approach from other environmental health statutes in that this regulatory scheme is not tied to the pathway of human exposure or the environmental medium but rather is directed at the risks of the chemical itself.

Record Keeping and Reporting by Manufacturers. Of critical importance to the operation of the act is Section 8(b), which provides for the publication and maintenance by the EPA of an inventory of all chemical substances manufactured or processed in the United States. Manufacturers and processors of selected chemical substances are required to report to the EPA the name of each chemical and its identity and proposed uses, estimates of production levels, a description of byproducts, adverse health and environmental data, and the number of workers exposed to such chemical substances.

Premarket Notification by Manufacturers. Manufacturers and processors of new chemical substances must give the EPA 90 days' notice prior to their manufacture or processing. This applies as well to a significant new use of an existing chemical substance. The notice must include all known data on health and environmental effects and must be available to the public for examination.

If the Administrator of the EPA finds that there is a reasonable basis for concluding that a new chemical substance presents or will present an unreasonable risk of injury to health or the environment, an order may be issued to prohibit manufacture of that substance.

Testing by the EPA. Under Section 4 of the act, the EPA may require the testing of a chemical substance to determine whether it may present an unreasonable risk of injury to health or the environment, if there is insufficient information for assessing the effects of the use of the chemical, and if testing is required to develop such information. Testing also may be required if a chemical substance will be produced in substantial quantities and it can be reasonably anticipated that there will be an extensive environmental or human exposure.

The purpose of the testing requirements is to screen the substances and mixtures for their potential for causing long-term health or environmental effects. Standards may be established for such health and environmental effects as carcinogenesis, mutagenesis, teratogenesis, behavioral disorders, cumulative or synergistic effects, or any other effect that may present an unreasonable risk to health or environment. Standards also may be established for such chemical characteristics as persistence, acute toxicity, subacute toxicity, and chronic toxicity. Particular methodologies such as epidemiological studies, serial or hierarchical tests, *in vitro* tests, and whole animal tests also may be specified.

The act also authorizes the establishment of an interagency committee that will advise the Administrator of the EPA concerning which chemicals should be tested. The committee may designate for testing, at any one time, up to 50 chemicals from its list of recommended substances. Within one year, the administrator must either promulgate testing requirements for those designated chemicals or publish in the Federal Register the reasons for not initiating rule making.

EPA Regulations against Unreasonable Risks and Imminent Hazards.   Under Section 6 of TSCA, the EPA may prohibit or limit the manufacturing, processing, distribution in commerce, use, or disposal of any chemical substance or mixture that is determined by the EPA to present an unreasonable risk of injury to health or the environment. In such a case, the EPA may require a manufacturer to do any of the following:

1. Label the chemical substance or any article containing the substance with clear and adequate warnings and instructions
2. Make and keep records of the processes used in manufacturing a chemical substance and conducting tests to assure compliance with any regulatory requirements
3. Give notice of any unreasonable risk of injury presented by the chemical substance to those who purchase or may be exposed to it, as well as to the public
4. Replace or repurchase such substance or mixture

In proposing such regulatory actions, the EPA must provide an opportunity for comments by all interested parties, an oral hearing, and, in certain instances, cross-examination. The act also has a unique provision for stimulating participation by public interest groups that allows the EPA to provide compensation, including reasonable attorney's fees and expert witness fees, to those unable to afford the costs of participating in these particular rule-making proceedings.

If a chemical substance or mixture contains a hazardous contaminant as the result of a certain manufacturing process, the EPA may order the manufacturer or processor to change the process or employ quality control procedures that prevent such contamination. Alternatively, the manufacturer or processor may be required to give notice to purchasers and to those who may be exposed to the hazardous contaminant as well as to the general public, and to repurchase or recall that product.

Exemptions.   The term "chemical substance" is defined broadly under the act, but a number of things are excluded from regulation, including pesticides regulated under the Federal Insecticide, Fungicide and Rodenticide Act; tobacco and tobacco products; nuclear materials regulated under the Atomic Energy Act; food, food additives, drugs, cosmetics, and devices regulated under the Federal Food, Drug and Cosmetics Act; firearms and ammunition subject to taxation under the Internal Revenue Code; meat and meat products regulated under the Federal Meat Inspection Act; poultry and poultry products regulated under the Poultry Products Inspection Act; and eggs and egg products regulated under the Egg Products Inspection Act.

The following chemical substances are exempt from the premarket notification requirements: (1) those listed on the inventory of existing chemical substances; (2) those produced in small quantities solely for experimental or research and development purposes; (3) those used for test marketing purposes; and (4) those determined by the EPA not to present an unreasonable risk. The first two are blanket exemptions, and the latter two must be sought on a chemical-by-chemical basis.

Litigation and Enforcement.   If a manufacturer files objections to an EPA order to prohibit manufacture of a particular chemical substance, the EPA must seek enforcement of the prohibition in federal district court. If a total prohibition is not necessary, the EPA may propose a rule that becomes immediately effective to limit the manufacture, processing, or distribution in commerce of the proposed chemical substance without having to go to court.

Under Section 7 of the act, the EPA may commence a civil action against any person who manufactures, processes, distributes in commerce, uses, or disposes of any chemical that presents an imminent and unreasonable risk of serious or widespread injury to health or the environment, to protect against such risk. In addition, the EPA also may bring an action to seize the chemical itself in such a case.

For purposes of administering the act, the EPA has broad authority to inspect any establishment in which chemicals are manufactured, processed, stored, or held before or after distribution in commerce.

Any person who fails or refuses to comply with any requirement of the act is subject to civil penalties assessed by the EPA, up to $25,000 per day of violation. The act also provides for criminal penalties of up to $25,000 per day of violation, imprisonment up to one year, or both. In addition, Section 17 of the act allows EPA to file civil actions in federal district court to seek injunctions to restrain activities prohibited under the act.

The Toxic Substances Control Act has a citizens' suit provision similar to those under the Clean Air Act, Clean Water Act, and RCRA. Section 20 of the act allows any person to bring suit, either to restrain a violation of the act by any party or to compel the Administrator of the EPA to perform any nondiscretionary duty required by the act.

In addition, under Section 21 of the act, any person may petition the EPA to issue, amend, or repeal a rule under the testing, reporting, or regulatory sections of the act. If the EPA takes no action or denies the petition, opportunity is afforded for judicial review in a federal district court.

Disclosure of Information.   One controversial provision of the act is Section 14, which sets ground rules as to the nature and extent of disclosure of information submitted to the EPA by chemical manufacturers, processors, and distributors. The chemical industry is highly competitive and quite protective about internally generated corporate information. On the other hand, there is strong public interest in the disclosure of all information that affects public health and the environment.

Section 14 of the act attempts to reconcile these divergent points of view by protecting from disclosure confidential data, such as trade secrets and privileged financial data, while authorizing disclosure of health and safety information submitted to the EPA under the act, except that such authorization does not extend to disclosure of manufacturing processes or the chemical proportions of a particular mixture. In addition, disclosure of even health or safety data may be withheld in certain cases under the Freedom of Information Act (for example, where a particular company is under investigation). Information other than health or safety data may be designated as confidential by the person submitting it.

Even information designated as confidential may be released, if the EPA disputes validity of the confidentiality claim or if disclosure of the data is necessary to protect health or the environment from an unreasonable risk of injury. However, the EPA first must give notice, in advance of the release, to the person who submitted the data. Such notice is not required for disclosure to federal officials responsible for protecting health or the environment or engaged in law enforcement, to government contractors where such information is necessary to the performance of their responsibilities, and to congressional committees that submit a written request.

Exports and Imports.   Exports and imports are subject to widely divergent treatment under the act. Imported chemicals are subject to all the requirements of the act, including the testing and premarket notification provisions. Exports, on the other hand, are generally exempt from the requirements of the act, except for those relating to reporting and record keeping under Section 8. The EPA, however, may elect to regulate or require testing of a chemical produced for export which may present an unreasonable risk to health or the environment of the United States.

Polychlorinated Biphenyls (PCBs).   PCBs were manufactured in the United States from 1929 until 1977. As noted in Chapter 3, they possess chemical and physical properties ideal for a broad range of commercial uses, but are hazardous to health at very low concentrations. Because of their chemical stability, they are very persistent in the environment and bioaccumulate in the fatty tissue of all organisms.

TSCA imposes specific regulatory requirements for PCBs. They now may be used only in a "totally enclosed manner" (such as in totally enclosed electrical equipment). Manufacture of PCBs after January 1, 1979, and processing and distribution of PCBs after July 1, 1979, is prohibited unless authorized by the EPA. As of July 1, 1984, the EPA had granted only few such authorizations, with certain health and environmental safeguards.

The Federal Insecticide, Fungicide, and Rodenticide Act (FIFRA)

History and Purpose.   FIFRA, as amended in 1972, 1975, and 1978, is the primary federal statute for regulating the manufacture, distribution, and use of pesticides. (Once a pesticide is discarded as a "waste," it becomes regulated under the Resource Conservation and Recovery Act.) Although FIFRA was enacted originally in 1947, pesticide regulation dates back to the Insecticide Act of 1910, which was principally a consumer protection statute designed to prevent the manufacture and distribution of ineffective, adulterated, and mislabeled insecticides and fungicides. FIFRA replaced the Insecticide Act in response to the proliferation of agricultural pesticides after World War II but preserved the predominant consumer protection theme.

This theme still remains — despite the substantial amendments to the act — but has been broadened somewhat in light of the increased public concern regarding the health and environmental effects of pesticides.

Under FIFRA, a "pest" is essentially any organism declared by the Administrator of EPA to be "injurious to health or the environment." A "pesticide" is, with certain specified exceptions,

> any substance or mixture of substances intended for preventing, destroying, repelling, or mitigating any pest, and . . . any substance or mixture of substances intended for use as a plant regulator, defoliant or desiccant.

This broad term thus includes fungicides, insecticides, herbicides, nematocides, rodenticides, disinfectants, desiccants, and defoliants.

Regulation and Classification of Pesticides.   Governmental premarket clearance and control of the estimated 35,000 pesticides now on the market is required as "protection against any unreasonable adverse effects on the environment." This includes the "economic, social, and environmental costs and benefits of the use of any pesticide." FIFRA requires all pesticide products sold or distributed in the United States to be registered with the EPA in a way similar to the premarket notification requirements of the Toxic Substances Control Act. The burden is on the registrant to prove that the product — when used as directed — will be effective against the pest or pests listed on the label, will not cause "unreasonable adverse effects" on the environment as specified in certain "risk criteria," and will not result in harmful residues on food or animal feed.

The EPA must classify a registered pesticide in either of two categories: general or restricted use. Classification for general use means that a pesticide, when applied as directed and "in accordance with a widespread and commonly recognized practice, will not generally cause unreasonable adverse effects on the environment." If such adverse effects can be prevented by imposing "additional regulatory restrictions," the EPA must classify the pesticide for restricted use. If the pesticide's use is restricted because it is acutely toxic to humans, it may be applied only by or under the direct supervision of a certified applicator. This authority to restrict use is extremely important in that it gives the EPA an option, for reducing pesticide risks, short of cancellation or suspension.

Under Section 6 of FIFRA, the EPA has the authority to cancel a pesticide registration if it is determined that its use causes "unreasonable adverse effects on the environment" or if it is mislabeled or misbranded. A registrant can appeal an EPA cancellation notice through a lengthy process that includes public hearings and ultimate judicial review. It took several years to restrict the use of such pesticides as DDT, aldrin, dieldrin, Kepone, heptachlor, and others. In order to prevent an imminent hazard during protracted cancellation proceedings, the EPA can suspend a pesticide registration, which immediately stops shipment of the product, pending completion of these proceedings.

The act also provides for the registration of establishments that produce pesticides. No person is allowed to produce any pesticide unless the establishment in which it is produced is registered with the EPA.

The EPA, by congressional consent and under an agreement with the Food and Drug Administration, is responsible for establishing tolerances for pesticide chemicals in or on raw agricultural commodities. The EPA also establishes tolerances for pesticides that may be considered as food additives under the Food, Drug and Cosmetic Act. Registration of pesticides cannot be accomplished unless food tolerances have been established or exemption from tolerances has been granted.

Amendments to FIFRA.   The 1978 amendments to FIFRA authorized the EPA to waive submission by the registrant of data related to the efficacy of the product. This represents an attempt to allow the marketplace, rather than EPA to police the effectiveness of pesticides, except where performance of the products has a direct bearing on public health. Pursuant to this policy, the EPA has waived submission of efficacy data for all pesticides except for rodenticides and disinfectants. The purpose of the 1978 amendments was to streamline the registration process.

Another attempt to achieve regulatory efficiency was made with the shift to "generic pesticide registration." In the past, registration entailed an examination of risk of each individual product. Generic registration, however, involves a single, comprehensive evaluation of risks and benefits of the technical material common to various similar products.

The 1978 amendment also provided for disclosure by the EPA to the public of the health and safety data supporting pesticide regulations. Other data, however, are specifically protected from public disclosure. As under the Toxic Substances Control Act, the EPA or other government employees — and those under contract to the government — who wrongfully disclose such data are subject to potential imprisonment or a fine.

Exemptions.   The registration requirement for pesticides is subject to three types of exemptions: experimental use permits; emergency uses, such as an anticipated pest outbreak for which no alternative is available to eradicate the pest; and state registrations for "special local needs." However, the EPA can disapprove state registrations.

Enforcement.   The EPA has the authority to enforce the provisions of the act by means of legal sanctions. The act prohibits the sale of unregistered, adulterated, or misbranded products; the use of any pesticide inconsistent with its labeling; and the production of pesticides in an unregistered establishment. Enforcement generally centers around monitoring industry compliance with product registration requirements and user compliance with label directions. This monitoring involves inspection of production establishments, marketplace surveillance, and sampling and analysis of pesticides. The enforcement sanctions are similar to those under TSCA: civil penalties, criminal fines, stopped sales, use or removal orders, recalls, seizures, and injunctions.

The 1978 amendments transferred to the states the primary responsibility for enforcing the pesticide use requirements for those states that can demonstrate they have adequate legal authority and implementing procedures to enforce these requirements. The EPA, however, has the authority to take independent enforcement action where states are unwilling or unable to enforce. In addition, the EPA can revoke all or a part of a state's responsibility for pesticide use enforcement if the state's program is found to be deficient.

REFERENCES

Druly, Ray M., and Ordway, Girard L. "The Toxic Substances Control Act." *Environment Reporter*, Bureau of National Affairs, March 11, 1977.

Environmental Protection Agency. Office of Public Awareness. "Everybody's Problem: Hazardous Waste." Washingbton, D.C.: EPA, EPA publication no. SW-826, 1980.

Jennings, Ralph (Chief, Toxic Substances Section, United States Environmental Protection Agency, Region IV). Interview with Keith M. Casto, September 8, 1981.

Rogers, William H., Jr. *Environmental Law.* St. Paul: West, 1977.

Stewart, Richard B., and Krier, James E. *Environmental Law and Policy.* New York: Bobbs-Merrill, 1978.

Index